The COVID Journals leaps off the page as a wonderful, compelling, important, and unique contribution to pandemic literature. Shane Neilson, Sarah Fraser, and Arundhati Dhara have curated a vital, energetic chorus of health care workers who use poems, visual art, and personal narratives to testify about their work, lives, and loved ones during the pandemic. A rich unmasking of those whom we too often herald as heroes but too rarely come to know, this anthology offers the reader an appreciation of the individuality, pain, love, humour, and creativity of Canadian health-care workers.

—LAWRENCE HILL, novelist and essayist

Just as stories have been central to our lives as human beings over millennia, they are also central to medicine. The narratives in *The COVID Journals* reframe health care as a human endeavor.

—PAMELA BRETT-MACLEAN, University of Alberta

The COVID Journals brings readers into an encounter with the pandemic that is as exceptional as it is ordinary.

—EMILIA NIELSEN, York University

The COVID Journals

Edited by
Shane Neilson,
Sarah Fraser,
and Arundhati Dhara

THE COVID JOURNALS

HEALTH-CARE WORKERS WRITE THE PANDEMIC

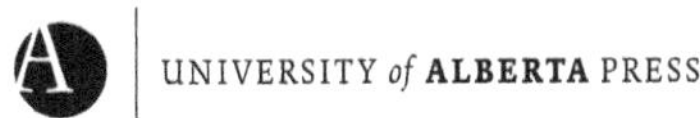

Published by

University of Alberta Press
1-16 Rutherford Library South
11204 89 Avenue NW
Edmonton, Alberta, Canada T6G 2J4
amiskwaciwâskahikan | Treaty 6 |
Métis Territory
uap.ualberta.ca | uapress@ualberta.ca

LIBRARY AND ARCHIVES CANADA CATALOGUING IN PUBLICATION

Title: The COVID journals : health-care workers write the pandemic / edited by Shane Neilson, Sarah Fraser and Arundhati Dhara.
Names: Neilson, Shane, 1975- editor. | Fraser, Sarah (Physician), editor. | Dhara, Arundhati, editor.
Identifiers: Canadiana (print) 20230169023 | Canadiana (ebook) 20230169074 | ISBN 9781772126815 (softcover) | ISBN 9781772126914 (PDF) | ISBN 9781772126907 (EPUB)
Subjects: LCSH: COVID-19 Pandemic, 2020- —Canada. | LCSH: Medical personnel—Canada. | LCSH: Medical care—Canada.
Classification: LCC RA644.C67 C68 2023 | DDC 362.1962/414400971—dc23

First edition, first printing, 2023.
First printed and bound in Canada by Houghton Boston Printers, Saskatoon, Saskatchewan.
Copyediting and proofreading by Joanne Muzak.

University of Alberta Press gratefully acknowledges the support received for its publishing program from the Government of Canada, the Canada Council for the Arts, and the Government of Alberta through the Alberta Media Fund.

Canadä

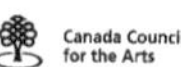

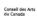

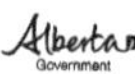

Contents

Preface

This book was born from the need to give voice to the unique experiences of health-care workers who had to deal with the greatest burdens of exposure during the COVID-19 pandemic, practitioners who did their jobs because they felt ethically obligated to do so, despite ambivalence. During the first few months of first-wave lockdown, Damian Tarnopolsky, a health-care writing instructor, first broached Shane Neilson with the idea of collecting an anthology of health-care narratives, poems, and art written by workers themselves as a good way to preserve that moment in time. Neilson and Tarnopolsky crafted and distributed a call for submissions and interacted with various medical journals to encourage them to direct material to the project. Soon after receiving the first dozen or so submissions, we decided that the project needed a more diverse editorial board. To that end, we reached out to the current co-editors of this volume, Sarah Fraser and Arundhati Dhara, to help attract a broader representation of submissions from various health-care fields. Sarah and Arundhati brought forward valuable contributions that substantially expanded this volume's scope, and provided keen editorial improvements upon the writing in this volume. Unfortunately, Damian had to step away from the project mid-completion, and in this preface we wish to acknowledge all the administrative, solicitation, and editorial work he performed, without which this book would not exist.

Before we summarize the contents of *The COVID Journals*, we'd like to itemize the benefits of writing out collective experience in the health-care realm. As Nick Pimlott, a senior physician in the collection, attests, over time there can be a loss of data concerning lived experience. In what is already referred to as an "infodemic"—the vast amount of information being generated in the scientific literature concerning the manifestations and particularities of COVID-19—there is more than a good chance that the dailiness of the lives of health-care workers, their challenges and satisfactions, can get lost. Perhaps especially so in the COVID-19 pandemic, one that has flattened out our chronologies to a digital perpetuity. As Pimlott shares in "A Journal of the Plague Year 2020," he was a trainee during the onset of the HIV pandemic and yet cannot recall what it was like, even as he remembers it as a formative experience in his life as a physician. Rather than letting pandemic life and the natural habits of memory shrink vivid narratives into flat categories and vagueness, we feel that collecting and preserving what otherwise might prove ephemeral is important.

Perhaps the individual contributors found a therapeutic benefit in terms of catharsis or processing of experience when writing out their individual narratives, poems, and diaries, or when making their art. We didn't ask them, because we are more interested in the benefit a collection of narratives, poems, and images can offer all of the health-care professions. Perhaps, in time, the collective memory will shrink to a slogan like THANK YOU HEALTH-CARE HEROES. Perhaps workers themselves will only remember that they served others and were glad to do so. Many may prefer not to look back on what has been a very difficult time. Others, though, need a balanced representation and reflection upon that difficult time, as related by someone doing similar work, to better understand their place in the past and their relationship to care in the present. Furthermore, public narratives often elide that which is difficult. The accounts herein, most of which are previously unpublished, do not shy from difficult testimony. This book can offer the curious, the nostalgic, and the suffering a useful touchstone for their experiences.

There are many other possible benefits of a repository of workers' lived experiences like the present volume. In this brief preface, we'll restrict ourselves to just one more. A book like *The COVID Journals* is intended to suggest a national experience for workers who live and practice in Canada. The stories are ours, at the least. Around the campfire, what listener would argue that the story is not better if it also "happened here"? For, if it happened here, it happened to an "us," acknowledging the disparities and inequities in Canadian economic systems.

• • •

The book itself is organized impressionistically. We initially segregated material into narrative, poetry, art, and diary sections, but ultimately decided that the full range of the experience could not be conveyed by making precise distinctions. The narratives in the section begin with Paul Dhillon's "Uncertainty," a metapoetic reflection upon whether, in the pandemic, there is no "resolution" to be had and that, if considered as a story, we are the pandemic's "antagonists," not the virus particle. Dhillon's narrated absence of patients in anticipation of the early nightmare projection of overwhelming numbers flooding ICUs sends the signal of what becomes a recurring theme. The art in *The COVID Journals* by Helen Tang and Tharshika Thangarasa considers iconography of the pandemic, especially as it relates to masks. The diary material in the book follows the legendary (albeit highly creative non-fictional) example of Daniel Defoe's *A Journal of the Plague Year: Being Observations or Memorials of the Most Remarkable Occurrences, as well Public as Private, which happened in London during the last Great Visitation in 1665*, as first published in 1722. These stories are moving because their initial intent was to document and heal, rather than to inform or inspire. Shan Wang protects her parents against contamination as she works in a care facility in Montreal during the first wave, becoming increasingly worn out as her time there progressed. In "A Journal of the Plague Year 2020," Nick Pimlott reflects on his regret of not documenting his experiences as he trained during the HIV/AIDS crisis. In response, he keeps meticulous notes of what happened over the first year of this pandemic, from finding small joys in cycling to deferring grieving for his father. In "Blowing Smoke in Your Ear," members of the African Nova Scotian community remove care from the hospital and place it squarely in the community. This story flips the notion of "health-care worker" on its head in a historic Black community that has been among those disproportionately affected by COVID in a province drawing international attention for low case numbers. Their experiences present a narrative of community-based care that takes over when formal health-care institutions don't deliver, and invites us to reflect on an expansive notion of love, faith, and family. As for the poems, they are a varied (formally and tonally) bunch. Elizabeth Niedra's hilariously sad "I Am Letting Myself Go" appears close to Governor General's Award–winning poet Tolu Oloruntoba's prose poem "The Sum of All Fears," which is anxious and hallucinatory. Monica Kidd is contemplative and analytical, reflecting on the surgical mask as icon using anaphora. Jordan Pelc's "Pandemic" ironizes the trope of science-based practice in the pandemic in free verse. Jiameng Xu's plaintive lyrics strike another note; the pulsed energy of Suzanne Lilker's "I'm No Hero" brings intertextual concerns to bear in dialogue with the television show *Scrubs*. Pam Lenkov's "Vicissitude" clinches a feeling we've all had in this pandemic, but in a hybrid form. The book concludes with the panoramically despairing, yet finding-joy-in-small-things, care-defiant "It's Hard Not to Slam a Fist on the Table When the Finish Line Keeps Lurching Further Ahead, or Third Wave." Candace de

Taeye's breathtaking poem is a metaphorically perfect conclusion to a pandemic that has taken much, especially breath.

• • •

Though this preface began in the past tense, of course we have not yet emerged from the pandemic. As we edited and revised the book, we kept changing the number of the pandemic wave we were in, waving goodbye to the previous number and waiting for the next surge. At the time of writing, COVID cases are once again on the rise, and the likelihood of even more infectious Greek letters by which we periodize our lives is high. Yet the writing in this book is primarily of the first and second waves, with an additional two contributors (Candace de Taeye and Tanas Sylliboy) covering more recent experience. The moment in which a storied killer was on the wind, changing how we were with one another so intensely, remaining home for the public good, wearing masks just like they did in sensational pandemic movies, not circulating with others in their homes and even at funerals—this is the moment we capture. The stories are ongoing but the stories in this book are, we feel, representative of the core experiences of health-care workers when things were at their most uncertain and fearful. And yet in those moments, there were still bits of joy to be had. This book is a record of the fear and joy health-care workers went through in the early months of the COVID-19 pandemic.

These narratives describe our new world, in which our faces and bodies (and thus our emotions) are masked. We broke bad news to our patients behind face shields and masks, so no one could see the expressions on our faces. It is unclear if this was better or worse than delivering such news virtually, mediated by screens. As personal protective equipment (PPE) was rationed and the physical examination discouraged, our identities and core function as care providers became more and more obscure. What is care if you can quite literally be nowhere near a patient? As we oscillated between various stages of lockdown, our primary social interactions became the hospital and social media.

Thus, we solicited and pondered over art. Reclaiming narratives as a radical vehicle for empathy, we hope readers will appreciate the stories as much as we did. The assembled prose, poetry, and visual narratives offer us alternative visions of COVID-19 pandemic. They tell us about how this pandemic *feels* for health-care workers who have watched it unfold. They are in turn tender, curious, and angry. They ask us to question what it means to care for someone.

Fight or Flight

1

The Ambivalent Health-Care Heroes of Pandemic Response, Canadian Edition

SHANE NEILSON

For Dr. Lorna M. Breen

Personal Disaster Medicine

A generation before mine—I'm Gen X, thanks Doug Coupland!—North American boomers had one dependable conversational topic other than the weather: *Where were you during the assassination of JFK?* For my generation, humanity's common conversation shifted to *Where were you when the planes hit the Twin Towers on September 11, 2001?*

Well, I was working in the Emergency Department of St. Clare's Hospital in St. John's, Newfoundland as a first-year family medicine resident, mired in the dead and ever-deadening middle of an internal medicine rotation. The waiting room at the Clare had a wall-mounted TV. News blared from the box, but to profoundly empty space. Rather than march to the emergency department for a remedy for what ailed them, as they usually did, that day Newfoundlanders preferred to stay at home to learn more about the American disaster.

Information hit consciousness like this: (1) the shock of a plane hitting the North Tower; (2) the shock of another plane hitting the South Tower; (3) the South Tower collapsing first, then the North; (4) two planes; (5) two buildings down; (6) Must Be Terrorists, Inc.

This prepackaged summary was quite unlike that which actual eyewitnesses were forced to piece together in real time:

> A mystery of a plane striking one of the Twin Towers—an accident?—what kind of plane?
>
> No, now a sinking realization of a deliberate act with the second strike.
>
> Shock: A tower collapsed? What? *They do that???*
>
> Eventual slippage into a ticking certainty that the second tower would collapse.

All of these action movie plot points I missed in experiential real time. I knew only the flat fact of them, all at once.

The COVID-19 pandemic is like the initial fog-of-war 9/11 sequence mentioned above, but in perpetuity. What's going to happen? What has happened? When will this be over? Is it over? Why isn't it over? What fresh hell will come? Will there be another lockdown? Another killer mutation? Do we need a booster shot? Why won't everyone get vaccinated? Another day, another evolving concern. Another conversation about what to do or what not to do. And, surely, the subject of a future conversation by billions who seek to reassure one another of their navigation of a mass trauma.

COVID Time

Despite my intense personal linkage of 9/11 with St. Clare's Hospital—reader, I feel at this moment soft hospital greens close to my body, a white lab coat on my back that carries too many little protective manuals, a prescription pad, nametag, reflex hammers, and stethoscope; I feel their encumbrance and stiffness—*there were no patients to see*. The hospital was quiet.

Emerg was still blocked, but owing to the lack of inflow, there were no new consults for me to process. I was free as a medical learner in a way I'd never been before during that deadening rotation and as I'd never be again for the remaining month. Even the floors were quiet, patients and nurses huddled around their screens and radios. I had nothing to do but sit in an empty waiting room and watch a television set suggest, over and over again according to the well-entrenched 24/7 news cycle loop, that a very great reckoning was coming: *War. War with those responsible. War. Warwarwar.*

There are many differences between my 9/11 medical experience and that of COVID-19. For example, COVID time prevents the culture from formulating a question like *What did you do when COVID first came to Canada?* because of the sheer achronological nature of the pandemic's time span, its seeming eternal stretch, perhaps only divisible in terms of waves and their subsequent lockdowns (first wave alpha, second wave alpha/beta, third wave delta, fourth wave delta, fifth wave omicron, sixth wave omicron BA2 subvariant, on and on, iterative waves). COVID has bequeathed us with a washed out and perpetual quality to life in the pandemic. *What were you doing when COVID ____?* etc. is more like a *What were we ALWAYS doing during COVID ____?* We're yet to pass it, to emerge from it. We're still caught in COVID time.

I see a continuity between 9/11 and COVID, however, as there always must be connection between traumatic historical events in one's life. That continuity finds inevitable expression through the lens of my physician identity. I analogize the 9/11 event as if the body sustained a trauma, perhaps a huge gash opening up on the leg.[1] Chronologically, though, 9/11 seemed to speed time up:

> War. War. War.
> Warwarwarwarwarwarwarterrorwarwarterrorterror.

COVID-19 is a far more mysterious affliction that has slowed time down, as if we exist in a fever dream where we wait for our fever to break, only to realize that, after glancing at the clock (again), just five minutes has passed since we last looked.

The continuity is substantiated by more than analogy. Consider 9/11 and 2020's empty emergency rooms, except this time not for a day and night, but *months*. Shared too is the idea that a reckoning was (and is) to come, but this time a reckoning for health-care systems threatened with a massive oversupply of critically ill bodies exceeding our capacity to ventilate them, underfunding of systems, disproportionate effects of catastrophes on marginalized people, racism and colonialism that permeate our systems, extractivism and late capitalism. And like the 9/11 disaster, reckoning possessed a double sense: not the "reckoning" *to come*, but rather the "reckoning" that *already was*. Planes hitting towers was, to one way of thinking, a radical political action to humiliate Americans and their smug foreign policy, one that successfully instigated war. COVID was a worldwide reckoning brought to us by globalist human economic activity and climate change.

COVID has forced many to face personal reckonings, too. For me, the professional valence at the start of the pandemic was this: after living a life in which so much has been sacrificed, lost, or denied because of non-normativity and madness, what should I do in this pandemic? Should I work from home due to the righteous explosion in virtual care options, or should I go in person to the clinic and do my job there? Perhaps most pertinent to that perpetual lens of my physician identity is this question: Is doing my job the simple contribution I can make to the "pandemic response"?

My answer now in the middle of the sixth wave is the same as during the first: maybe.

We Could Be Heroes, Just for One Day

In April 2020, deep into the first lockdown, I began to weary of "health-care heroes" talk, of video clips showing fire and rescue personnel circling hospital buildings in demonstration of solidarity; of national coffee chain signs splashing their tickertape with the letters H-E-R-O-E-S to attract the attention of motorists as they raced down Brock Road to enter into Guelph.

Whenever a nation refers to heroes, I thought, *it needs cannon fodder.* That is a very old lesson, but always a good one. The best example I can think of using a Canadian poet is John McCrae, whose "In Flanders Fields" was used on recruitment and fundraising posters for the Dominion and beyond in the First World War. McCrae, of course, was a soldier himself, also a physician, born in Guelph.

The rhetoric of pandemic heroism was only going to increase, however, so much so that health-care writing pedagogist Damian Tarnopolsky and I devised a creative writing workshop for health-care workers that pushed against this very idea. The workshop ran in the summer of 2020 and, as I suspected, none of the participants were feeling particularly heroic. Everyone seemed exhausted, drained, and yet happy to do work that was relatively pointless.

Driving home to Oakville from that workshop one night, I saw another coffee chain sign celebrating the heroism of first-line responders. By now, the term had broadened to include grocery store workers, supply chain personnel, basically anyone crushed under neoliberalism's Gucci boots, anyone who needed some social capital to substitute for the material kind.

And for some strange reason, my mind turned to the story of Dr. Lorna M. Breen, an emergency doctor at New York-Presbyterian Allen Hospital who died, according to her father, because of her work during COVID. "She tried to do her job and it killed her," he said. He added, "She was truly in the trenches of the front line...Make sure she's praised as a hero, because she was. She's a casualty just as much as anyone else who has died" (Watkins et al. 2020).

Trenches.
Front line.

Hero.
Casualty.

From there, the beginnings of a poem etched into my mind as I sped towards Trafalgar Road. Before long, I was in my driveway, about to enter Pandemic House—my irreverent christening of my home—and have an hour with my children before bed, before taking a heroic sleep and assumption of the next day's heroic mantle.

But as I was about to succumb, a notification buzzed on my phone. That night, the Ontario Medical Association held a town-hall-style meeting on Zoom concerning physician wellness during the pandemic. Something in the back of my mind, the self-protective little wizened troll that whispers *Take care* from under my mental bridge, a monster that, against type, tries to keep me alive—he whispered, *Get the laptop, you should watch this.*

I caught the proceedings late, but early enough to catch a crucial minority report. An older physician panelist, one who had practised during the severe acute respiratory syndrome (SARS) crisis, said, "I know everyone dislikes this 'hero' business. But I have to let you know something. In the last pandemic, you know what? Rather than talk of heroes, the public discriminated against us. I know physicians who were avoided and shunned because of their work. People were terrified that they would catch a killer disease from us. Maybe we should be less dismissive of the 'hero' stuff. It could be worse."

Receiving compelling opposition to what until then was an unopposed, fixed belief of mine was liberating. As sleep came on, I resolved to verify the esteemed panelist's experience with a quick review of the literature the next day.

We Were Heroes

It turns out that the senior colleague was correct. One needs not to leave the current century in order to discover stigmatization of health-care workers in a pandemic; perhaps even more close to home in a literal sense is the fact that the epicentre of the SARS pandemic in North America was Toronto. In "Impact on Health Care Workers Employed in High-Risk Areas during the Toronto SARS Outbreak," the authors relate that "HCWS [health-care workers] reported instances of stigmatization, which often included their family members" (Styra et al. 2008, 178). In addition, 60 per cent of survey respondents "indicated that friends and neighbors avoided them, while 36% reported that people avoided their family members because of concerns of contracting SARS" (180). Isn't this the same hero cohort, though, as the current pandemic?

"Heroism" is merely the public face of a positive current. As Sanjeet Bagcchi puts it in *The Lancet Infectious Diseases*, "healthcare workers and patients who have survived COVID-19 are facing stigma and discrimination all over the world" (2020, 782). In a statement made on March 18, 2020, the World Health Organization (WHO) noted that "some healthcare workers may unfortunately experience avoidance by their family or community owing to stigma or fear. This can make an already challenging situation far more difficult" (2). Bagcchi mentions that in May 2020, "a community of advocates comprising 13 medical and humanitarian organizations including, among others, the International Federation of the Red Cross and Red Crescent Societies, the International Hospital Federation, and the World Medical Association issued a declaration that condemned more than 200 incidents of COVID-19 related attacks on healthcare workers and health facilities during the ongoing pandemic" (2020, 782). What I suspect is different with COVID-19, though, is the coincident heroism rhetoric alongside recognition of stigma. Bagcchi describes the multi-agency condemnation as follows: "The recent displays of public support for COVID-19 responders are heartwarming, but many responders are nevertheless experiencing harassment, stigmatization and physical violence" (782). The most obvious reason why we have heroism rhetoric now is because the public desperately needs health-care workers. SARS was largely a hospital-acquired infection; almost half of those who acquired the disease were health-care workers. Social ostracism and stigma in this case were an ancient means to contain the threat. With COVID-19, however, the distribution was wider, just as with the 1918 influenza pandemic. Medical historian Howard Markel explains that social scapegoating was "not all that loud" then because "the pandemic spread so rapidly and ubiquitously among all sectors of American society (especially among those 20–45 years of age)" (2007, 52). Rather than harass people needed in the fight, the productive social response was to valorize the fighters of COVID, enlisting all the overnight heroes that could be metaphorically press-ganged. Grocery bag stuffers, shelf-stockers, personal support care workers, nursing home clinic aides, doctors, and nurses now had heroic stuff, but only for as long as it would take for life to return to normal.[2]

Forced to pick between heroism and stigma, I'd love the privilege to choose neither; but this is not how the world works. *I chose heroism then*, I thought after I had made my confirmation, and began another literature search, hoping to discover more about what the experience of "heroism" has been in pandemics past.

Heroes Get Sick and Die

One of the commonalities in pandemics throughout history is the fact that health-care workers are disproportionately affected by the burden of illness. In "Past as Prologue," David Heymann of the WHO summarizes a limited selection of the late twentieth and early twenty-first centuries' viral outbreaks in which health-care workers figured centrally in morbidity, mortality, and disease transmission: Ebola in the Democratic Republic of Congo and smallpox in England. He soon settles on a true pandemic with H2N2 in 1957, in which "52 percent of unvaccinated health workers in New York City and 32 percent of unvaccinated health workers in Chicago became infected themselves" (2007, 34). He adds, "The lesson is clear: Health workers and caregivers are inevitably on the front line in a pandemic" (34). And of course, let us not forget SARS in 2003.

Though I dislike military metaphors in medicine and have written a good deal to discourage their use, I must acknowledge that Heymann has a case, one that extends its application to the COVID-19 situation. The "front line" metaphor has merit—just as it did with the first responders who rushed into the Twin Towers to rescue people. As different as I'd like medicine and war to be, the closeness of the variables and their relations are inescapable. I get claustrophobic when thinking of firefighters rushing up the North Tower stairs, just as I do when I see, as is inevitably repeated at least once on network television on the anniversary of September 11, George W. Bush repeat the following words as if we are all frozen in time once more: "Every nation, in every region, now has a decision to make. Either you are with us, or you are with the terrorists."

Does this sound like a pandemic of power to you, too? A single moment of a decision and a forever of consequences? Bush's equation has never left, existing as a kind of temporal stasis ever since; the anniversary of 9/11 reminds us that in some everywhere, during some everywhen, people died; and for that, other people must die. War, because first responders died. War, because the definition of the "front lines" was redrawn to the home front, just as COVID has redrawn the front lines of care to screens.

Forgive me; my mind is wandering in grief. And in such grief, my mind thinks according to lyric. I suppose this is my own no man's land.

Lyric Essay Fragments on Medical War Memorials

In Sofia, the capital of Bulgaria, there is a monument. Set on a simple square base, a series of slabs rise in a tapering fashion to a terminal ark-like cap. Inscribed in the slabs are 529 names. The entire site is called the "Doctor's Garden" and is situated behind the SS. Cyril and Methodius National Library. The monument was completed in 1884 in memory of doctors and nurses who died while working for the Russian Red Cross during the Russo-Turkish War (1877–1878).

• • •

The Spanish-American War Nurses Memorial sits on the grounds of Arlington National Cemetery in an area informally called the "Nurses Section." The war of 1898 was the first featuring nurses as a dedicated unit. None of the 153 deaths were due to direct combat. Most came as a result of infectious disease, including yellow fever. The memorial itself is a large grey rock, with wave-like grooves cut into the upper half as if the rock were moulting its layers. At the very top is a sculpted Maltese cross, a symbol derived from the original mark of the Knights Hospitaller, an ancient order devoted to the care of the sick, poor, or injured. The United States suffered 1,691 casualties in that war and 260 fatalities, but far more personnel became ill due to typhoid, malaria, dysentery, and yellow fever. In a review of Vincent Cirillo's *Bullets and Bacilli: The Spanish-American War and Military Medicine*, Emil Gotschlich (2005) writes that because of infectious disease "less than one-quarter of the Army that had gone ashore on June 22, 1898, remained fit for service" by the beginning of August.

• • •

WWI dead: There are various estimates. Some are as low as just under ten million and others as high as sixteen million.

• • •

Pandemic dead of 1918: There are various estimates. Some are as low as twenty million and others as high as fifty million.

• • •

In "Influenza in Canada: A History," Niall Johnson wonders if John McCrae "succumbed to what may well have been influenza on January 28, 1918, at Wimereaux near Boulogne, France" (2018, 5). McCrae suffered from lifelong asthma and the generally accepted thinking of both his biographers, John Prescott and Diane Graves, is that he died from pneumonia and meningitis. But as Johnson and many others explain, cause of death is tricky to attribute; deaths to influenza were routinely misattributed at the time. The first official cases of influenza in France were noted in April 1918, with the first similarly clear case of influenza "ever" occurring in at a military base in Kansas in March 1918; yet the true nature of some limited pre-pandemic outbreaks cloud the picture. As Johnson writes, current thinking (the same that exists around COVID, in which the virus, based on modern testing, has been proven to have been circulating globally before the first wave was apparent) suggests "herald waves" and "pre-seeding of epidemics" make it "entirely plausible that John McCrae was one of the first Canadian victims of this historical pandemic" (Johnson 2018, 5).

• • •

In November 1984 the stolid and functional Canadian Military Medical Services Memorial was unveiled in Borden, Ontario. There were 1,394 names originally inscribed in the monument, beginning with the Boer War (in which McCrae fought). The memorial required modification in 2009 to allow for the addition of new names of fallen health service members. In between the entries Pte McCoy AE and Cpl McCreary SE, the name LCol McCrae J can be found.

• • •

In May 2015 the Remember Flanders memorial, commissioned by the Royal Regiment of Canadian Artillery, was unveiled on Green Island Park in Ottawa. To those who don't know McCrae's incredible backstory, his memorialization by the Royal Regiment of Canadian Artillery might seem to be militaristic jingoism. Yet McCrae not only served as brigade-surgeon to the First Brigade of the Canadian Forces Artillery, he was also second-in-command. He could—and did—give combat orders and soldiered as a gunner. To me, the statue is heartbreaking because it feels so lifelike, in kin with McCrae the man. He looks like he's about to hop off his log, his back ramrod straight in the military style; and yet it's also as if he's about to start writing a poem in the notebook in his left hand.

• • •

A sequential listing of non-duplicated search results of "War Memorial Hospital" using Google's engine:

> War Haldimand WMH in Dunnville ON. Sault Ste Marie WMH in Marie MI. Great WMH in Perth, Ontario. Uniting WMH in Waverley, Australia. Gosport WMH in southern England. Tarporley WMH in northwestern England. Nakuru WMH in Kenya. Purley WMH in South London, England. Burnside WMH in South Australia. Brampton WMH in northwest England. St. Andrew's WMH in Brisbane, Australia. Arran WMH in Scotland. Andover WMH in southeast England. Colonial WMH in Suva, Fiji. Let us not forget the veterans memorial hospitals and the soldiers memorial hospitals.

Wars disappear from our public mind just like pandemics do. However, the physical structures of the hospital remain. As much as these memorials entail the celebration of victory and place a capstone on sacrifice, they also sit atop our collective souls and say: *You built me in part because you have wars.*

Fighting and Flighting

Running through the historical record concerning physicians' behaviour during pandemics is a moral theme in which physicians are both expected to stay and fight against disease and also not to refuse treatment to the ill. All of this is understandable. I too desire tales of the medical greats remaining in their plague- and pestilence-ridden cities, ministering to the ill tirelessly. As is the way of things, the comportment of physicians has been variable in individual cases, albeit in the main creditable. According to medical historian Daniel Fox, for "most epidemics for which records survive, most physicians seem to have treated most of the patients who sought their help" (1988, 5). There are, of course, notable exceptions.[3] One of my medical heroes is Galen, so I looked up his behaviour in Rome during the Antonine plague in 163 CE.

Gasp. Galen fled to Pergamum. And he wasn't alone: many physicians over the centuries left their cities for the countryside during plague season. For example, Thomas Sydenham ran from London in 1665. Fox writes of "some leaders of the profession in Philadelphia and New York during outbreaks of yellow fever in the eighteenth and cholera in the nineteenth centuries" who did the same (1988, 5). "In addition, many physicians who did not flee reportedly refused to visit patients who were acutely ill" (5).[4]

The ethical basis for some of these decisions *seems* lacking. How could wealthy doctors leave their practice for the tranquility and relatively infection-free countryside? How could they abandon their patients? Tracking history with a moral lens can be trouble, however. As Fox points out, some physicians followed their *patients* to the countryside. President George Washington, Secretary of State Thomas Jefferson, Secretary of War John Knox, and Secretary of the Treasury Alexander Hamilton all followed the advice of Benjamin Rush to leave Philadelphia (then the seat of American government) in 1793. Some physicians left because of reasonable fears of death, following through on the same recommendation they made to their patients. Do we blame the many people living under COVID who took their families and left large metropolitan areas in North America for the countryside, partly to avoid infection?

On the other hand, the ethical basis for other decisions *is* lacking. Wealthy doctors were generally less inclined to treat the poor. As a result, pandemic history is peppered with stories of immigrant physicians promised citizenship should they agree to function as plague doctors for an affected city. The modern parallel in the COVID time frame are immigrant health-care workers in the US, who—cue martial metaphors in this piece in the *Journal of Hospital Medicine*—"are on the front lines in the fight against COVID-19 in the United States, accounting for 16.4% of healthcare workers amid this pandemic" (Mathews and Malik 2020, 505). Looking at the specific cohort of hospitalists, a whopping 32 per cent are international medical graduates. As the article states, "many of these doctors—more than a third of those practising in this country who graduated from international medical schools—have visa restrictions that limit their ability to work in communities with the greatest need" (505).

A parallel can be drawn to the behaviour of certain physicians who did remain in their cities during the pandemic. Fox writes of "local physicians" who used surgeons to "care for plague patients," surgeons being afforded a less-than status in Europe all the way up to the nineteenth century (1998, 6). He continues, "The physicians recommended that the surgeons shout the 'quality, sex, and condition of the patient and stage of illness' from an open window to a physician at a safe distance, who would then shout back a course of treatment" (6). A modern-day metaphor of virtual care is somewhat applicable, albeit one that once again must consider the advantages of privilege and class.

Advocacy for refusal of treatment of non-vaccinated individuals during the COVID pandemic have been made by several physicians on social media, a truly pestilential line of thought given that many vaccine-hesitant people are marginalized individuals. This kind of othering found its modern nadir during the HIV pandemic. In "The Morality of Refusing to Treat HIV-Positive Patients," Mitchell Silver quotes a *New York Times* article covering the case of Dr. W. Dudley Johnson, a "distinguished heart surgeon" who "had refused to operate on two patients because they were positive for HIV, the virus associated with AIDS" (1989, 149). Mitchell's article quotes several surveys with distressingly high numbers of physician respondents who would refuse to treat HIV-positive patients.[5] As a result of the prevalence of these opinions, medical bodies in North America enforced a duty to care.

But then there are real heroes, ones that happen to double as my *personal* heroes. My all-time favourite, Dr. Benjamin Rush (mentioned briefly earlier), made Herculean efforts during the yellow fever epidemic of 1793 in Philadelphia, seeing up to one hundred patients a day at its height. Yet Rush's example embodies one of the unintended side effects of heroism. As comes up fairly often in the articles about physician response during pandemics, the problem is often not so much underserving the poor as overtreatment with phlebotomy and purgatives—part of the armamentarium of now-antiquated "heroic medicine."[6] Of note in Rush's story is that he became ill himself, and that three of his five assistants died of yellow fever, demonstrating the common theme of the burden of exposure for health-care workers.

When interviewed in the *Journal of the American Medical Association* (JAMA) in 2020 by Angel Desai, the medical historian Dr. Howard Markel opines, "The worst thing about the last act of every epidemic or pandemic I've ever studied is something I call global amnesia. We tend to forget about it, and the political actors go on to the next issue" (2020, 2119). It is my hope—as well as that of the co-editors—that this book makes some small resistance against forgetting what it was like for health-care workers in Canada during the COVID-19 pandemic.

Notes

1. The American response to the cut was less a suturing and more a self-seeding of the wound to make it suppurate, but I digress.
2. At the time of revision, October 12, 2022, normal time has yet to resume.
3. My history here is abbreviated and non-scholarly. "Big man/woman" history is of course misleading; Fox explains that the history of physician response during pandemics is more complicated, involving medical ethics discourses operative at the time as well as civic/public health responses to pandemic crises that resulted in contracted services. And yet "big man/woman" history is the kind that inspires our imaginations most readily. Perhaps this approach can be resuscitated in the following sense: in *America's Forgotten Pandemic: The Influenza of 1918*, Alfred Crosby says the pandemic wasn't one huge mononarrative but rather "thousands of separate stories" containing huge differences in effects and outcomes (2003, 66). So it is with the tales of physicians.

4. In “Plagues throughout History and the Doctors Who Treated Them,” James H. Brien (2014) mixes the martial rhetoric with compassion when he writes, “It is my contention that there were unsung heroes who stayed on their job, attending to their patients, knowing that they might acquire the disease and knowing that if they did, they might die. In some ways, this is worse than war. At least in war you are fighting an enemy with the same fears as you, and you can see him, and you have a fighting chance. When you are dealing with invisible enemies—even if you could see them, you would not know how to kill them.” Fear, anxiety, war, mortality, killing—heroes. This is the grim thematic intersection.

5. Silver provides a lengthy philosophical discourse to arrive at a conclusion that supports the treatment of HIV-positive people because the risk of infection is very small, but the final rationale remains distressingly close to hero rhetoric: “Developments may require a revision of that judgement. It may turn out that caring for HIV-positive patients, or at least certain kinds of care, does run a serious risk of infection. In that case the treatment of HIV-positive patients would no longer be a duty, it would be a heroic act. But that time is not now and given present knowledge it seems not on the horizon” (1989, 157). Tina Turner belted it best: “We don’t need another hero. We just need to find the way home.”
6. “Heroic medicine” refers to a kind of therapeutic philosophy that advocates for extreme purging, bloodletting, and inducement of sweating in order to shock the body back to health.

References

Bagcchi, Sanjeet. 2020. “Stigma during the COVID-19 Pandemic.” *The Lancet Infectious Diseases* 20 (7): 782. https://doi.org/10.1016/S1473-3099(20)30498-9.

Brien, James. 2014. “Plagues throughout History and the Doctors Who Treated Them: Part I.” *Infectious Diseases in Children.* October 22, 2014. https://www.healio.com/news/pediatrics/20141203/plagues-throughout-history-and-the-doctors-who-treated-them-part-1.

Crosby, Alfred W. 2012. *America’s Forgotten Pandemic: The Influenza of 1918*. 2nd ed. Cambridge: Cambridge University Press.

Desai, Angel. 2020. “Twentieth-Century Lessons for a Modern Coronavirus Pandemic.” *JAMA* 323 (21): 2118–19. doi:10.1001/jama.2020.4165.

Fox, Daniel M. 1988. “The Politics of Physicians’ Responsibility in Epidemics: A Note on History.” *The Hastings Center Report* 18 (2): 5–10. https://doi.org/10.2307/3562420.

Gotschlich, Emil C. 2005. Review of Vincent Cirillo, *Bullets and Bacilli: The Spanish-American War and Military Medicine*. *The Journal of Clinical Investigation* 115 (1): 3-3. https://doi.org/10.1172/JCI24100.

Heymann, David. 2007. “Past as Prologue?” In *Ethical and Legal Considerations in Mitigating Pandemic Disease: Workshop Summary*, edited by Stanley M. Lemon, Margaret A. Hamburg, P. Frederick Sparling, Eileen R. Choffnes, and Alison Mack, 33–44. Washington, DC: National Academies Press. https://www.ncbi.nlm.nih.gov/books/NBK54171/.

Johnson, Niall. 2018. “Influenza in Canada: A History.” *Defining Moments*. https://definingmomentscanada.ca/wp-content/uploads/2018/06/From_Bad_to_Worse.pdf.

Markel, Howard. 2007. “Contemplating Pandemics: The Role of Historical Inquiry in Developing Pandemic-Mitigation Strategies for the Twenty-First Century.” In *Ethical and Legal Considerations in Mitigating Pandemic Disease: Workshop Summary*, edited by Stanley M. Lemon, Margaret A. Hamburg, P. Frederick Sparling, Eileen R. Choffnes, and Alison Mack, 44–60. Washington, DC: National Academies Press. https://www.ncbi.nlm.nih.gov/books/NBK54171/.

Mathews, Benji K., and Manpreet Malik. 2020. “Immigrant Physicians Fill a Critical Need in COVID-19 Response.” *Journal of Hospital Medicine* 15 (8): 505–06. https://doi.org/10.12788/jhm.3473.

Silver, Mitchell. 1989. “The Morality of Refusing to Treat HIV-Positive Patients.” *Journal of Applied Philosophy* 6 (2): 149–57. https://www.jstor.org/stable/24353380.

Styra, Rima, Laura Hawryluck, Susan Robinson, Sonja Kasapinovic, Calvin Fones, and Wayne L. Gold. 2008. “Impact on Health Care Workers Employed in High-Risk Areas during the Toronto SARS Outbreak.” *Journal of Psychosomatic Research* 64 (2): 177–83. https://doi.org/10.1016/j.jpsychores.2007.07.015.

Watkins, Ali, Michael Rothfeld, William Rashbaum, and, Brian Rosenthal. 2020. “Top E.R. Doctor Who Treated Virus Patients Dies by Suicide.” *New York Times*, April 27, 2020. https://www.nytimes.com/2020/04/27/nyregion/new-york-city-doctor-suicide-coronavirus.html.

World Health Organization. 2020. “Mental Health and Psychosocial Considerations during the COVID-19 Outbreak.” Bulletin, March 18, 2020. https://www.who.int/docs/default-source/coronaviruse/mental-health-considerations.pdf.

Uncertainty

PAUL DHILLON

> *Uncertainty is an uncomfortable position, but certainty is absurd.*
>
> —VOLTAIRE, letter to Frederic II, King of Prussia, April 6, 1767

What if there is no resolution?

What if we are the antagonists?

Every epic story has a protagonist, antagonist, an inciting action, conflict, and resolution.

By many and most accounts, every human has now been touched in some way by the inciting action. The theory at the time held that this action took place in an ignominious wet Wuhan market. A quiet scene, methyl-mercaptan-scented water drips from scaled lifeless fish atop crushed ice, a simple cough perhaps, and then the story truly begins.

Even those infants just born of the tumultuous months of 2020, bereft of words to tell their story, miss moments with a father's touch in the first seconds of birth, of life. COVID-19, our protagonist, touches us all.

He, she, COVID-19's amorphous manner makes it difficult to pin him or her down. While we rush, headstrong, to learn so much about our protagonist in the first few chapters of this story we perhaps fail to pause and reflect on the antagonist's response. What will it be? And how will the antagonist's decisions affect and make consequence of the protagonist?

Early days of the pandemic caused quick and calculated reflection on my experiences working in a viral hospital, during the Ebola epidemic in 2015. Far more virulent, on an individual level, but controlled and not a pandemic. Memories of rubber boots sloshing in chlorine-impregnated water with the remains of viral particles and mortality beyond compare. Were we seeing it again? Italy? New York? Belgium? Did we need to be scared? How bad could it possibly be?

Then the inconsistencies began. The questions were raised. Why here? Why not there? Why? Why? Why?

The human mind has a magical manner in which to fill in gaps in our stories, in our histories, and in our future. As rational as we like to believe we are, another story, we fear the unknown and search, seek, and story our way through that muddling unknown. Stories of cure, of the quick fix, rapidly filled in the gaps of rationality that were based in a basement of fear.

Similar to basements being a place of refuge during evening onslaughts from the Luftwaffe we once again had to retreat to our homes. Curtains drawn, twitched opened only for a check on the dangerous behaviours of those we were trying to protect by staying in our homes.

My experience was complicated with the need to be at work during the COVID Ides of March. As a member of the team tasked to create the surge hospital facility in Vancouver, British Columbia, we were engulfed in the maelstrom at a local level. We still wait. The predicted savage single storm has now become a season.

The season, I believe, this will be the lasting impact of this pandemic, the inconsistency and uncertainty, the wait for the climax, the conflict that has not arrived, leaving resolution an unfinished and unkempt beast. A season not a storm.

Over the course of days and weeks an empty windowless cavern in the Vancouver Convention Centre was transformed from a place of mass gathering, a taboo now, to a place of potential convalescence and healing, an unintended and unimaginable forethought.

Teams were assembled, organic and flowing with a joint unity of purpose. A clear mission and task with orders rested alongside an understood greater good. Planning for weeks, work for simply eight days, and it was thus. Almost biblical, from an empty room rose a hospital. Replete with hundreds of beds, oxygen concentrators, and Red Cross supplies.

Late evenings, walking to my sequestered hotel room during the hospital build was eerie. Streets normally full to the brim or overflowing with weekend revelry were barren in the downtown core. Screaming cheers were replaced with silence. It was post-apocalyptic. You could imagine a virus had swept through and the mortality was the cause of the silence, but in fact it was the opposite. It was the living causing the deep silence. An incredible collective moment, imposed, yet believed and trusted. Evening would briefly shatter this silent interlude with a cheer to the health-care workers, then expanded to the "front line," another ode to war that still was on pause. Waiting for the conflict, the moment to achieve victory, and the wait went on. And still goes on.

Build a hospital, and hope they don't come. But was that true?

The stress, the preparation, and the micro *internecine* battles that occurred across Canada in medical institutions from the rural hospital to the gargantuan mega-hospitals as traditional boundaries and silos were broken, shattered, and cobbled together again into defences against a single foe.

Patience, patience, patience—while waiting for patients, who would never arrive. Victory?

Yes, victory but pyrrhic? There lies a victory in that fact that there were no patients in the surge hospital but there was no closure for those who worked on the opening. Without the impending conflict we wait in a suspended state. No fire to forge and test our creation. It's a beautiful pregnancy with no birth and all the drama that it entails.

Is a hospital with no patients ever really a hospital?

We sit and await the conflict, the opening to allow for a closure. That vast, vapid emptiness of the hospital with beds made, never unmade leaves a gap in the story, missing chapters that if left unwritten signal victory outside the walls, not within.

There is still hope, and sometimes in a story, all we have is hope as we turn the pages.

The protagonist faces significant obstacles—namely, billions of us. All we control is the antagonist's actions.

We still wait, wait, for that fevered crucible, the moment Blackadder goes forth, but in the interminable battle against COVID-19, that is a moment that arrived with a bang, but likely leaves with a whimper.

The Sum of All Fears

TOLU OLORUNTOBA

No stranger to enacting genocide, Winston Churchill once said, "Why, you may take the most gallant sailor, the most intrepid airman or the most audacious soldier, put them at a table together—what do you get? The sum of their fears."

In a way, he was right. They feared their own deaths dealt by the industrial-military complex. Where

> The sum of all positive integers in all nuclear sequences is an infinity of grief.
>
> The sum of all positive and negative integers is the zero-rim of the abyss.
>
> Nike is the goddess of the defeat of factory workers.
>
> The global south is a human head held below water.

You can find graphesthesia there, too; read the writing on the dusk. No Chinook copters interrupted the forced and final pilgrimage from Chibok, roads shivering under pickup tracers, analysts watching the infrared feed, the phosphorescent alarms of eyes rising like gooseflesh from the dark. Read the writing of your skin crawl: the rising bond—belt, corset, choker, blindfold. Read the ransom note: the boa is regurgitating you, but into another boa. Examine what could be your empty hands.

When you find the most gallant sailor, the most intrepid flight captain, or the most audacious soldier, you would have found the fundamental fears, the pincer movement of the same war. The sum of their war crimes is death. Specifically, the fear of death.

Haptic sharkskin suits, the arctic palpitations of their emergence from water with cyclopean night vision, their silencer barrels telescoping, ready-aim-fireant-swarming, pillaging banks of the sleeping; *that* is anxiety sensitivity.

When witch-eye drones with blue-bellies wear the sky, the glint of which wedding parties see too late, the flint of which air force analysts with superior hand-eye co-ordination hurl before their lunch break; when the gnat cloud of Starlink and DARPA satellites are the eyes of Argos Panoptes co-opting the full stratosphere for vision, the fear of negative evaluation is watching over you.

Siege warfare depended on attrition, the dwindling grain, the sleepy lookout. Under the iron cloud of pestilence, we may have faltered, resigning the drawbridge to the trebuchet, the ballista, the unaccountable fist, bones crushed to dust under the mailcoat of siege engines. But that came later. The emissary was already within, by then. A good besieger can cow with the one hand, undermine walls with the other: to mine beneath the earthen ramps, and deliver the singular saboteur. These tactics can depend on the element of surprise: that call when you're far away at work after they got your child. Read the ransom note: the ambulance is on its way. No, the child is unresponsive. Your heart, outside your body these three years, in the body of another, is unresponsive.

The fear of marine boots launched through the splintering door of your body; this fear, is the fear of injury.

The sum of all fears is that of the great unknown, specifically the fear of death.

Specifically, the death of a child.

Specifically, the possible death of a child one is twenty-six kilometres away from, racing toward in a friend's car on the TC-1, butterfly-pinned to the passenger seat, dialing and redialing to see if the ambulance has arrived at the school, if the child is now conscious.

The circuit breaker of her body, sensing the furnace it was becoming, dimming her wakefulness; the seal-team hands of hypoxia smothering her lungs; the jackboot march of her seizures; those were the pincer movements of an invading force.

Perhaps the pandemic began in December 2019, when I launched myself, a missile seeking my daughter's heat, hoping to arrive on time.

References

Carleton, R. Nicholas. 2016. "Fear of the Unknown: One Fear to Rule Them All?" *Journal of Anxiety Disorders*, no. 41, 5–21. https://doi.org/10.1016/j.janxdis.2016.03.011.

Clancy, Tom. 2002. *The Sum of All Fears*, vol. 5. New York: Penguin.

Cunningham, Anna. 2016. "Why Has Nigeria Failed to Rescue the Chibok Schoolgirls from Boko Haram?" *CBC News*, April 14, 2016. https://www.cbc.ca/news/world/nigerian-schoolgirls-boko-haram-1.3535324.

International Churchill Society. 2013. "Churchill on War." *Finest Hour*, no. 134 (Spring 2007). Posted on June 10, 2013. https://winstonchurchill.org/publications/finest-hour/finest-hour-134/churchill-on-war/.

Kelland, Kate. 2020. "A Study Reveals That Coronavirus Had Spread around the World by Late 2019." *World Economic Forum*, May 7, 2020. https://www.weforum.org/agenda/2020/05/coronavirus-spread-around-world-2019-study/.

A Journal of the Plague Year 2020

NICK PIMLOTT

Another plague year would reconcile all these differences; a close conversing with death, or with diseases that threaten death, would scum off the gall from our tempers, remove the animosities among us, and bring us to see with differing eyes than those which we looked on things with before.

—DANIEL DEFOE, *A Journal of the Plague Year*

COVID-19 is the fourth pandemic to directly affect my medical career. The first was the AIDS crisis, which began with the report of the first cases in 1981 in the *Morbidity and Mortality Weekly Report* from the Centers for Disease Control in Atlanta. This was during my first year as a graduate student at the University of Toronto, and one of the first journal clubs I organized for students in my department was to discuss papers speculating on the cause, which at the time was unknown.

I started medical school in 1987. By that time, the virus that caused AIDS, the human immunodeficiency virus (HIV), had been sequenced. When I entered the hospital wards as an intern in 1991, no treatment had yet been found. By the time I began my career as an academic family doctor at Women's College Hospital in Toronto in 1994, effective treatment had been found. My last patient with HIV died from it in 1997. A small number of men with the virus in my practice are still alive and well today. Yet HIV remains a serious illness affecting over thirty-nine million people in the world, two million of them children under age fifteen.

One of my regrets is that I didn't keep a journal in those critical years of my family medicine residency looking after mainly young men with HIV/AIDS. It was a difficult time to learn to be a doctor, but a historic one with many lessons learned that we can apply today. My memories have faded of that time. Since I became the scientific editor of *Canadian Family Physician* in 2009, I have learned to keep a journal of ideas for editorials. In this pandemic I decided to keep a plague journal, even if intermittent and, as my daughter likes to say, "random," to keep the memories and the lessons alive in the post-COVID-19 pandemic future. These are some of my entries during that first, intense six months of the pandemic.

January

Sunday, January 26

This evening my family and I took my mother-in-law, Marlene (and father-in-law, Bernie), out for a birthday dinner at a modest Italian restaurant of her choice close to their home. In the background above the bar a television was on and Global news reported that a man with the first suspected case of severe acute respiratory syndrome coronavirus 2 (SARS-COV-2) or COVID-19 had been admitted to Sunnybrook Hospital, close to where we live. The dinner mood was light and festive, but mine was darkened by the news. Memories of the months when in 2003 SARS blighted our work and either killed or made gravely ill some of our friends and colleagues came to life. But public health leaders expressed no concerns, behaving as if we had nothing to worry about for the moment.

Monday, January 27

The National Microbiology Lab in Winnipeg confirms that a man in quarantine in Sunnybrook Hospital is Canada's first documented case of the new coronavirus SARS-COV-2. This may turn out to be one of those "where were you moments" for a younger generation—like "Where were you when Neil Armstrong landed on the moon?"

February

Crickets! No diary entries in February. Like everyone else, I was either oblivious to the threat, or quietly and anxiously waiting for all hell to break loose.

March

Wednesday, March 11

The World Health Organization declares a global pandemic of SARS-COV-2.

Friday, March 13

Kathy and I decide to drive to our cottage near Parry Sound, Ontario, three and a half hours north of the city. We think with a coming lockdown, it will be the last time we will be able to visit for a long while. It's not an easy journey and we arrive at dusk. Since we go up in winter so infrequently, the one-kilometre road into our place is not plowed. It means walking in and pulling all our supplies (including drinking water) on a large, black plastic toboggan, the kind used by snowmobilers. In the cold and fading light, only our dogs, Labrador Millie and springer spaniel puppy Dixie, seem to be enjoying the hike.

The late winter snow underfoot is hard on top, but soft below, and we keep breaking through, making for an awkward half-hour walk in (in summer it takes about ten minutes). We arrive to find that the power is out and we can't find out why or when it will be restored from the Hydro One app on our phones. We get the woodstove going to heat the upper-level kitchen, dining and living area, and sleep on the pull-out IKEA sofa bed close to the fire. We will regroup in the morning and decide if we are going to be able to stay.

Saturday, March 14

Kathy and I wake up in the cold and there is no sign that the power will be back anytime soon and now she is feeling sick—sore throat and the beginning of a cough. We quickly pack up and make the trudge to the van heading back to the city. Later, after her symptoms get worse, and she was left with a lingering malaise that lasted two weeks, we will wonder if she had COVID-19. A couple of weeks earlier she had been to a scientific conference in Ottawa with participants from around the world.

Tuesday, March 17

It's St. Patrick's Day and since the snow has made way for spring early, I have decided to ride my bike to work as often as the weather will allow. That way I can avoid public transit and driving to work.

My first five or six years in the family practice clinic at Women's College I used to ride my bike to work almost every day. Then, one morning, as I was turning left on Southvale Drive onto Bayview Avenue I was rear-ended by a driver turning right against a light from Moore Avenue. I was knocked to the ground, but unhurt, and in my rage and fear I leapt to my feet and started banging on the driver's side window, yelling. Then I recognized the driver—Peter Worthington, former publisher of the *Toronto Sun* newspaper—and he looked frightened. I got back on my bike and rode to work, but that would be the last time for several years. Around that time a star University of Toronto researcher around my age, and, like me with three young children, was killed by a City of Toronto truck while bike commuting home.

For my first ride down, I leave a bit early and take the long route—into Serena Gundy Park and down the valley along the Don River and climb up to Wellesley Street at the bottom of

Rosedale Valley Road. The enterprising owner of the corner store at Parliament and Wellesley Streets has plastered handmade signs on the storefront window in bright pink and neon green advertising masks, gloves, and hand sanitizer for sale. Along Wellesley Street to Bay Street, usually bustling in the mornings, there are few cars, no cyclists and no pedestrians.

Wednesday March 18

Today was my first evening urgent care clinic of the pandemic (each family doctor in our practice does one of these clinics roughly every month). Midway through the evening, I see a young woman in her early twenties who has just returned from volunteering in sub-Saharan Africa. With her travel history she is presumed at risk for having COVID and she has some minor symptoms. I was anxious and flustered having to gown, glove, mask, and wear a face shield for the first time since SARS in 2003, and felt angry and resentful towards this affluent young woman, putting me at risk. I am not proud of feeling this way, as in the previous SARS and AIDS pandemics, such feelings were unknown to me.

Tuesday, March 24

Getting into an enjoyable routine of cycling to work down the Don Valley. My ride begins with a rapid descent of about three hundred metres with a sharp left-hand turn and over a metal bridge that spans the West Don. This morning someone has strung the signs "Hope" and "Love" from a tree to the bridge stanchions, one sign on each side. Briefly, I feel touched by the sentiments, but having reread parts of Daniel Defoe's *Journal of the Plague Year*, the skeptic in me wonders how long such sentiments will last.

Friday, March 30

Today I was invited to a meeting with leaders at the hospital to discuss a paper recently published in the *British Medical Journal* (*BMJ*) by Trish Greenhalgh describing a way to remotely look after COVID-19 patients at home using video visits. The paper is based on first principles since no one has any significant experience providing such care yet. We decide to launch a similar program.

April

Thursday, April 23

It is the end of the day routine "huddle" for the CovidCare@ Home Clinic. We now have over forty-five patients in the program and the question arises—How long should we follow patients? Some patients are eleven or twelve days since the onset of their symptoms and are only mildly ill—Can we discharge them? One of my colleagues provides a cautionary tale. Earlier today a previously healthy eighty-year-old man with mild symptoms "crashes." EMS is called and he is transferred to hospital. The unspoken is now spoken—the disease is unpredictable and we may not be able to prevent severe illness or death no matter how closely we follow people.

Friday, April 24

This morning is my first "virtual" clinic—I haven't spoken to many of my patients since the pandemic was declared. By the end of the morning, the visits are starting to feel like reunions with long lost friends.

Saturday, April 25

Met by phone with the third-year resident who has been one of the real leaders in staffing the CovidCare@Home clinic. We are beginning to write up the first case series to share our experiences, since most of what we know about COVID-19 at the moment comes from hospitals where patients are sicker. So far, in spite of lack of experience, the people we are looking after are doing well.

One of the main differences with this pandemic versus the AIDS crisis and SARS is that because of my age (higher risk for complications) I've been kept from seeing any patients in person. It feels odd. Dissonant. Like reports of the current plague are from another country. An article in today's *Globe and Mail* by history professor Timothy Neufeld compares plagues—this one he rates as a "meh" compared to the 1918 influenza pandemic and the Black Death. Strangely, no mention of the AIDS pandemic, which has killed over forty million people since the 1980s. Not sure I have much confidence in Professor Neufeld's assessment of our predicament.

Sunday, April 26

Began reading Roderick Haig-Brown's 1951 essay collection *Fisherman's Spring* earlier this week, a spring ritual for the past few years. Reading it just about makes up for the fact that I never get out fly fishing on the opening day of trout season. His essays seem like dispatches from a simpler time, yet in the 1950s and '60s pollution of rivers by industry was probably at its worst in the twentieth century and he was an activist. My two favourite essays are "The Maculate Purist" and "The Unexpected Fish." Maybe they speak to an aging doctor. Six weeks in I'm missing face-to-face care of my patients and being able to perform a physical exam and put it all together. The zealots think the pandemic will put paid to most in-person care and both the ritual and craft of the physical exam, already under siege for a generation from the evidence-based medicine movement. So, like Haig-Brown's commitment to fishing with the fly only, I find myself a maculate purist wanting to practice medicine as a manual craft the way I was taught. "The Unexpected Fish" reminds me of the unexpected diagnosis, a strange mixture of pleasure and sadness in it—the thrill of picking up a serious illness early, but awareness of the difficulties and the suffering by your patient in the days and weeks ahead. The smartest kid in the class meets real-world suffering.

May

Wednesday, May 6

Today I worked in the CovidCare@Home clinic with Anne Xia, a very thoughtful first-year family medicine resident. It was her first virtual COVID clinic and not surprisingly she lacked confidence, but did a great job. In between video visits we discussed the pandemic, and previous ones. One topic that came up was scapegoating and prejudice in plagues. During the AIDS pandemic I witnessed the prejudice against gay men. Acquaintances would ask me if I was afraid to look after patients with HIV and AIDS. By the time I was seeing patients in hospital as a student, it was known how HIV spread and that simple precautions protected health-care workers. Walking one morning to her palliative care rotation at St. Michael's Hospital in April someone on the street starting yelling at her to go back to her own country. This is her country and as a young doctor on the front line she is looking after all of us.

Friday, May 8

Today would have been my Dad's eighty-fourth birthday. It has been six and a half months since he died in hospital in Victoria, BC, from complications of surgery to remove a large tumor from his bladder. The pandemic has delayed grieving since last autumn my brothers, sister, and I had planned a memorial gathering at my brother Iain's home later in May. He wanted us to scatter his ashes on the Red River, which Iain's home backs onto. His ashes remain in a box on a cabinet in my basement. Today is the first time in over twenty-five years that I have not sent him a gift of a book to read. When will we be able to gather again?

Saturday, May 16

The cover story of this morning's *Globe and Mail* features the headline "46 Ways Our World Is About to Change"—a collection of short pieces by experts on what the world will be like post-pandemic. Sadly, many of the articles were about how we will be returning to a more inconvenient and expensive version of our previous way of life.

As an example, an air travel expert writing about how flights will cost twice as much and lineups will be four or more hours long as security staff swab people for COVID-19, but no imagining a very different life in which air travel once again becomes a luxury, as it was when I was growing up in the 1960s and '70s. In his book about the climate crisis, *The Democracy of Suffering*, Canadian philosopher Todd Dufresne estimates that more than 95 per cent of human-induced carbon emissions have occurred since about 1969, which is around the time, for example, that cheap air travel was beginning to become accessible to the average middle-class citizen in high-income countries.

Sunday, May 17

It's Victoria Day weekend and normally we would be up north to open the cottage, but cottage owners in the city where COVID cases are highest have been discouraged from going by local mayors and health authorities. So, we're staying put.

There was a great article in the April 20 edition of the *New Yorker* that I finally got around to reading today—a profile of Anthony Fauci by Michael Specter called "The Good Doctor." Fauci has been the head of the National Institute of Allergy and Infectious Diseases for almost forty years and has served six presidents. As Donald Trump mismanages the pandemic in the US, aided and abetted by several Republican governors, Fauci is once again turning out to be a kind of hero, as he ended up being during the AIDS crisis. At the beginning of the crisis he was hated by AIDS activists like Larry Kramer, but he listened and learned from them—for example, about the limits of the conventional medical approach to drug approval, which was slow and cost lives—and created a parallel fast track for AIDS treatments. Now Fauci says, "in American medicine there are two eras: before Larry (Kramer) and after Larry. There is no question in my mind that Larry helped change medicine in this country." For his part, Kramer, who spent years in a constant rage at Fauci, now calls him "the only true and great hero" among government officials during the AIDS crisis.

I was reminded while reading this that Specter also wrote a 2013 *New Yorker* profile about another famous American physician—Mehmet Oz—called "The Operator: Is the Most Trusted Doctor in America Doing More Harm Than Good?" Oz has been a long-time purveyor of quack treatments as a family physician friend, Mike Allan from the University of Alberta, and his colleagues showed in a brilliant article published in the *BMJ*. Recently, Dr. Oz has apparently been advising Donald Trump. Both Fauci and Oz are quintessentially American figures, the one representing so much that is good about the US, the other the kind of hucksterism and self-promotion that he shares in common with the president. No wonder Trump can't stand Dr. Fauci.

July

Friday, July 16

Kathy and I were supposed to start our summer holiday at Wahwashkesh tomorrow, but this evening around seven o'clock we called her parents to check in before leaving in the morning. Her father, Bernie, who is eighty-eight years old, has been having discomfort in his legs at night—so much so that for more than a week it has been waking him up. He tells Kathy that he took a couple of her mother's gabapentin capsules (which she takes for peripheral neuropathy pain in her arms and legs), but they haven't been helping much. Kathy's mom, Marlene, rats him out and says he has also been unable to walk from one end of their condominium to the other without getting short of breath halfway. I get him on the phone, and he sounds like he might be having trouble finishing longer sentences as well. He has had no chest pain, no palpitations, or other acute symptoms so I arrange to go and see him first thing in the morning. I'm pretty sure we will be delaying our holiday plans.

Saturday, July 17

Just after 8:30 in the morning I headed over to Kathy's parents' place with my black, leather doctor's bag in hand. Bernie and Marlene got this bag in Florence almost thirty years ago on a trip to Italy and gave it to me as a medical school graduation present in 1991. It's held up rather well over the years of doing home visits though the corners are frayed and the clasp doesn't close as tightly as when new. As I make my way up to their tenth-floor condo on the elevator it strikes me that I haven't examined a patient in almost three and a half months.

It turns out that Bernie is in bad heart failure, but the reason isn't clear. He has gained almost eight kilos of retained fluid, causing his shortness of breath, his legs to swell, and that "pain" he was feeling at night in bed. His vital signs are stable and although he has long-standing atrial fibrillation, his heart rate, while still irregular, is well-controlled. It's off to Sunnybrook Hospital to the Emergency Department to get him more thoroughly assessed. It's clear that the changes have been going on for several weeks (and we have been unable to see them in person until recently). It makes me wonder how many older people like Bernie are getting into trouble as they avoid (or are unable) to see their doctors, one of the anticipated outcomes in the first wave of a pandemic. Since late March my colleagues and I have been calling our older patients, especially those living alone, for a brief check in.

I'm allowed to sit with Bernie until he gets called in to be seen by the emergency doctor. After that I have to leave and we have to keep in touch by phone, a scenario which is being played out in hospitals across Ontario in which families are not allowed to be by the bedside of their sick, sometimes dying relatives.

Sunday, July 18

There have been lots of newspaper articles and blog posts about the healing power of nature in a pandemic and how nature is "rebounding" as human activities like driving and airline flights have ground to a halt. Close to home that seems to be true. Our house is under a busy flight path, but now when we sit in our backyard there is respite from man-made sounds. On a walk with Millie this past Thursday evening, I saw a cormorant patiently fishing from a log in the West Don near our place. Today Kathy and I took Millie for a two-hour walk in nearby Glendon Forest. We saw a grey catbird, a pair of American redstarts, and a pair of rose-breasted grosbeaks in the woods. Further along the path was a female snapping turtle likely going to lay her eggs, but trapped by all the pedestrians.

I discovered the healing power of nature long ago during the AIDS crisis—as an intern I took up fly fishing. When you fish you lose any sense of self and all its burdens, so focused on the water, the lie of the fish, the hatching insects, and the graceful movements of casting do you become.

Saturday, July 24

While on holidays I haven't been writing much in my journal, replacing writing with fly fishing.

This was the first clear night in a few days, so at eleven o'clock Kathy and I went out on the dock with our eldest son and his girlfriend to see if we could catch a glimpse of Comet NEOWISE. There it was in the northwest night sky just below the Big Dipper and above the tree line behind our cottage. I could just see it in my peripheral vision with the naked eye but got a spectacular view of it in all its brightness with my binoculars. NEOWISE will next return to Earth in about six thousand years. With the climate crisis already upon us, and most of our leaders (and the public) in denial, will there be any humans left then to see it?

August

Saturday, August 1

This morning while on holiday at the cottage I woke to news that an essay I had submitted to the *Globe and Mail* had been published on the front page of the Opinion section. Although

I knew it had been accepted, I did not know when it would be published, so this comes as a bit of a surprise. Just after ten in the morning my friend Kelly MacDonald calls from Winnipeg to congratulate me and to offer to be my "agent" since he speculates I might become the next Ian Brown with paid-for writing junkets on which I will need a travelling companion. I point out that as far as I know, Ian Brown isn't getting rich as a writer and it's unlikely I'll be able to give up my day job. But we have a good laugh about it.

The essay is about physicians literally losing touch—the ability to see and examine patients—during the pandemic. It was inspired by Roderick Haig-Brown's lovely essay "The Maculate Purist," drawing parallels between the practice of medicine and the skills of fly fishing.

Saturday, August 22

This morning I read a great article published August 7 in *The Atlantic* by journalist Kurt Andersen. It's called "College-Educated Professionals Are Capitalism's Useful Idiots." The subtitle is "How I Got Co-opted into Helping the Rich Prevail at the Expense of Everybody Else." It's hard to sum up briefly, but it's about how he and his college-educated fellow journalists contributed through their uncritical reporting to the decline of America's working and middle classes and the rise of income inequality. It's also about the inexorable march of capitalism to replace expensive, skilled human labour with machines and the economic and social consequences. Until recently, doctors like me have felt immune to the forces of "mechanization" of our skilled labour, but with the rapid shift to virtual care during the pandemic, it feels like we have opened the door to just such a change in medicine. Will doctors in the pandemic turn out to be big tech's useful idiots?

Tuesday, August 25

Now four and a half months into providing virtual care to my practice, it is beginning to wear thin even though, as an academic family doctor, I am only "seeing" patients two days a week. I realize that I spend the best part of each day in the clinic sitting in front of a computer screen simultaneously on the phone. Gone is the usual liminal space between each patient encounter allowing time to change scenes, reflect on the visit and stretch one's legs. By day's end I feel like I work in a call centre, with the main difference, as a waggish colleague said, that "No one hangs up on you."

It is also lonely. Most of my family medicine colleagues are doing their clinical work from home as one of the goals during the pandemic has been to reduce everyone's risk of exposure to COVID-19. The hospital, however, mandated that staff directly employed by them (like the secretaries and nurses in our clinic) had to work in person. As the associate chief of our team, I felt from the beginning that I should be on-site to check in on those people so physicians would at least have a presence. Some of the themes that have emerged for me about family doctors' work during the pandemic are raised by Wendell Berry in the essay "Economy and Pleasure," about the impact of the industrialization of farming, part of a collection titled *What Are People For?* and include the loss of community and the loss of a deeper pleasure in work.

September

Saturday, September 5

It looks like fly fishing might undergo a similar renaissance during the pandemic as it did after the release of the 1992 Robert Redford–directed film *A River Runs Through It*, based on the Norman Maclean novella. In today's *Globe and Mail* Ian Brown has an essay called "Quite a Catch: Finding Solace in Fly Fishing."

The best parts of the essay are the middle and the end. In the middle he writes about his crash course fly-casting lesson from Rob Cesta, owner of Drift Outfitters fly shop in downtown Toronto, and his fly-tying encounter with Chris Krysciak when he dropped by the shop one day. Drift is in the unlikeliest place for a fly shop—across from Moss Park in an area frequented by drug dealers, sex workers, and the homeless. Rob and Chris are as unpretentious and generous about their love of the sport and encouraging newcomers as the location of their shop.

After a day fly fishing on a river for bass Mr. Brown concludes, "Fly fishing, I suddenly thought, is very, very hard. It is especially hard to do well, and impossible to do perfectly... it humbles you into admitting you know much less than you think, that what you do know is often useless and that you need the help of others." Many of the same things could be said about medicine during these early days of a global pandemic. In the face of a brand-new disease, once again we have realized that as physicians, we know much less than we think, although some of the things we know about treating other conditions, like severe asthma, for example, led to the most effective early treatments of COVID-19. With the rapid early shift to virtual care, it has been impossible to practice medicine perfectly, but in a time of crisis, it has been possible to practice "good enough" medicine.

References

Anderson, Kurt. 2020. "College-Educated Professionals Are Capitalism's Useful Idiots." *The Atlantic*, August 7, 2020. https://www.theatlantic.com/ideas/archive/2020/08/i-was-useful-idiot-capitalism/615031/.

Berry, Wendell. 2010. *What Are People For?: Essays*. Berkeley, CA: Counterpoint Press.

Brown, Ian. 2020. "Quite a Catch: Finding Solace in Fly-Fishing." *The Globe and Mail*, September 6, 2020. https://www.theglobeandmail.com/canada/article-quite-a-catch-finding-solace-in-fly-fishing/.

Dufrense, Todd. 2019. *The Democracy of Suffering: Life on the Edge of Catastrophe, Philosophy in the Anthropocene*. Montreal and Kingston: McGill-Queen's University Press.

Haig-Brown, Roderick. (1964) 2014. *Fisherman's Spring*. New York: Skyhorse.

Greenhalgh, Trisha, Gerald Choon Huat Koh, and Josip Car. 2020. "COVID-19: A Remote Assessment in Primary Care." *BMJ*, no. 368, m1182. https://doi.org/10.1136/bmj.m1182.

Korownyk, Christina, Michael R. Kolber, James McCormack, Vanessa Lam, Kate Overbo, Candra Cotton, Caitlyn Finley, et al. 2014. "Televised Medical Talk Shows—What They Recommend and the Evidence to Support Their Recommendations: A Prospective Observational Study." *BMJ*, no. 349, g7346. https://doi.org/10.1136/bmj.g7346.

Pimlott, Nick. 2020. "In a Pandemic, Physicians Are Losing Touch with Patients. How Can They Strengthen Ties to Their Craft?" *The Globe and Mail*, August 1, 2020. https://www.theglobeandmail.com/opinion/article-in-a-pandemic-physicians-are-losing-touch-with-patients-how-can-they/.

Specter, Michael. 2013. "The Operator: Is the Most Trusted Doctor in America Doing More Harm Than Good?" *The New Yorker*, January 27, 2013. https://www.newyorker.com/magazine/2013/02/04/the-operator.

Specter, Michael. 2020. "How Anthony Fauci Became America's Doctor." *The New Yorker*, April 10, 2020. https://www.newyorker.com/magazine/2020/04/20/how-anthony-fauci-became-americas-doctor.

What I Will Not Doff

DIANA TOUBASSI

Our rings are on the kitchen counter. We removed them, my husband and I, when we realized they were potential vectors. They have waited there since, in a corner by the window, in the alternating sunlight and moonlight. They count for us what we struggle to count for ourselves: the days of the pandemic.

I still remember slipping off my band. I remember, too, a vague intuition of the gesture's meaning. We are responsible, dedicated physicians, I encouraged myself. We take seriously our duty to patients, want to eliminate even the smallest chance that we could transmit the virus on our rings.

But...what a price this is to pay.

• • •

"They're a couple," David told us.

My husband, an internist, was reviewing the list of patients admitted to our hospital's COVID ward. I'm a family physician, about to begin my deployment to the very same ward. Rachelle, the bright, tough internist who will co-attend with me, joins us by phone for the handover. I wonder if she shares my anxiety about taking over the following morning.

"She's 92; he's 97," David said. "She came first. Dyspnea, oxygen-dependent. He seemed initially to be holding his own at their retirement home, but then developed anorexia and malaise."

"So he's admitted also?"

"Yes. They're together, husband and wife. They wanted to be in the same room."

I looked at him.

"The family knows she may pass soon, but they wanted them together."

I heard Rachelle's breath over the phone.

"And..." David hesitated. "Their daughter is sick now, too."

The following morning, we embarked on our rounds in "the new way," one of us pushing a mobile workstation, reviewing results and typing notes, while the other donned and doffed PPE to assess patients in their rooms. The unit's charge nurse and a young, ebullient social worker travelled with us.

Our first visit with the elderly couple revealed Mrs. I. to be much more severely afflicted. In contrast, her husband appeared relatively well. He spoke very little, saying only "no" and shaking his head when directly questioned or offered food or drink. But otherwise, he was stable. He needed neither oxygen, nor fluids, was able to ambulate to the bathroom independently, and had more or less normal bloodwork.

I called their daughter after our rounds and tried to prepare her.

"Thank you, doctor," she said. "I'm sorry, it's a lot to process, especially when I feel so ill myself."

I marveled at her composure in the impossible situation.

"If she passes," she continued, "please tell him. Because I can't be there now, please tell him on my behalf. And then help him to FaceTime our family. He will want to see his grandkids."

I promised we would do as she asked.

On our fourth day on service, Rachelle shook her head when she exited their room.

"She's very close now."

I nodded.

We began to walk to our next patient's room, a middle-aged man who seemed destined for the ICU, when we were intercepted by a nurse. I struggled to identify her under her goggles, face shield, and mask; the paraphernalia intended to shield us from the virus seemed also to alienate us from one another. I didn't recognize her until I heard her voice.

"Mrs. I. has passed," she informed us. "Will you come back to declare her?"

I observed Rachelle as she carefully donned her PPE to enter their room again. Out of care for the process, we were always silent when one of us was donning or doffing. It occasionally struck me that there was something sacred about the transformation—the ritual we performed so many times a day to protect ourselves, our patients, our families. We tried not to relax, not to get complacent about observing the numerous steps in the sequence, to pay them proper respect.

After inspecting the cuffs of her gloves and the neckline of her gown, I nodded, permitting her to enter. I stood at the doorway, flanked by our charge nurse on one side, our social worker on the other.

There were two before, I thought. Now there is one.

Rachelle kneeled at Mr. I.'s bedside and leaned in. I didn't hear her words, but I saw his stillness.

Or...there was one before, and now there is half.

He said nothing, asked no questions, made no gestures.

She waited a bit, then exited and doffed.

None of us said anything for a short while. Whatever words needed speaking were spoken by the silence.

"I'll bring him the iPad in a few minutes," our social worker finally said. "I can help him call his family and I'll stay as long as they need."

I smiled thinly, out of gratitude, not yet accustomed to the mask that concealed half my face. As we walked again toward our next patient's room, I looked back at Mr. I., his door open, his eyes watching us.

What must he see? I wondered. A homogenous army in blue, each soul indistinguishable from the other, all unknown to him, all removed from the chasm that has just opened in his life. What must it be, to have his wife of decades, lie absent in the bed beside his, as he bucks up against his own sickness and frailty and utter aloneness. What can be left for him now?

In the ensuing days, Mr. I. ate less and moved less. I continued to call his daughter daily, to update her and ask for guidance. What would he want for his care? What do you want for his care? Still coughing and unwell, she asked me to buy his favourite from the lobby food court.

"Give him dumplings, please, Doctor. Or fried chicken. He'll eat it all, I promise," she pleaded, through her own sputtering breathlessness. I did as she asked, but to no avail. He simply shook his head, gently, insistently, and turned away.

I tried to see into him, to conceive the person and the life before me. But the protective layers on my face obscured both my literal and figurative view. He was vague. He couldn't (or wouldn't) tell me his story. And when I tried to imagine it, I felt only the love and worry in his daughter's voice, and then deep, deep sorrow.

As he continued to decline, we arranged for his daughter to visit—a logistical challenge, requiring special dispensation and considerable co-ordination. Our charge nurse intercepted her at the hospital entrance, assisted her to don her own PPE, then escorted her directly to his room, from which she was forbidden to venture until her departure the following day.

Mr. I.'s daughter called me after this visit, perhaps appreciating for the first time the reality of his situation. We agonized jointly over his disposition. It wasn't clear to either of us how much of his ongoing deterioration was due to COVID, and how much, the enormity of his loss, the impossibility of coping with its magnitude at his advanced age, in his compromised state.

Mr. I. passed a few days after Rachelle and I completed our deployment. I wanted to call his daughter again, one last time, but worried that she may find such a call intrusive.

Not long after, a friend of my husband's telephoned him.

"Your name, and Diana's, are in the paper," he told him.

We read the paired obituaries together.

"He grew up on the family strawberry farm."

"She worked as a hairstylist, seamstress, and letter sorter."

"During World War II, the family farm was taken by the Canadian government and the family was sent to a work camp in Alberta for five years where they picked sugar beets."

"He gave his energies to his family, especially his grandchildren whom he adored, and taking care of his wife in her later years."

"She seemed at peace at the end of her life and her final words were 'arigato' (thank you)."

"He died from complications related to COVID-19, and after losing his wife nine days earlier."

They filled in the empty spaces, these colours and fragments of life, gave form and substance to the couple we had cared for. I thought of Mr. and Mrs. I. in their formless gowns and nondescript beds, ashen and stationary, separated from their loved ones, disconnected from their past, isolated from everyone and everything known to them—save for one another, a few feet apart, in an old Toronto hospital room.

I thought of all the virus had taken from them—their independence, their health, and ultimately, their lives. But I thought also of all it had failed to take: the care and devotion of their family, and their connection—their unshakeable connection—to one another. I heard Dylan Thomas: "Though lovers be lost, love shall not; / and death shall have no dominion."

I sat quietly for a while, thinking about the I.s—this family that had intersected with mine, this couple that had been cared for by a couple. David watched me rise then, and walk into our kitchen, where our wedding rings still perched on the windowsill. I looked down at mine for a bit as it glistened in the sun, then picked it up. I can remove it before my next shift, I reassured myself, and slipped it on. The best of life will not be taken.

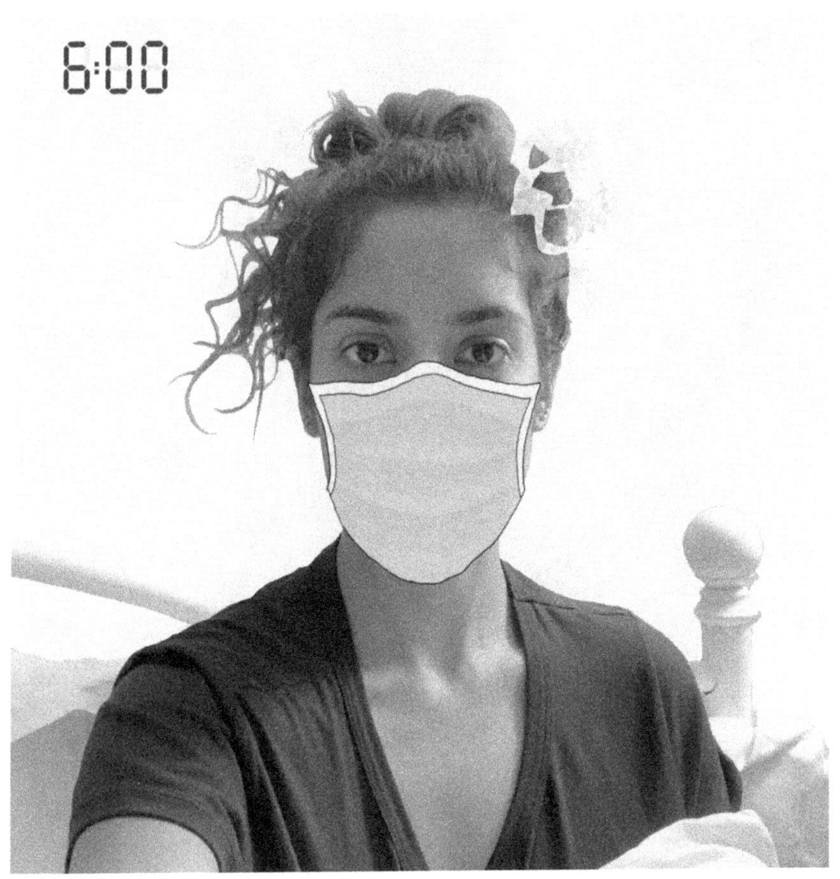

Workday by Tharshika Thangarasa.

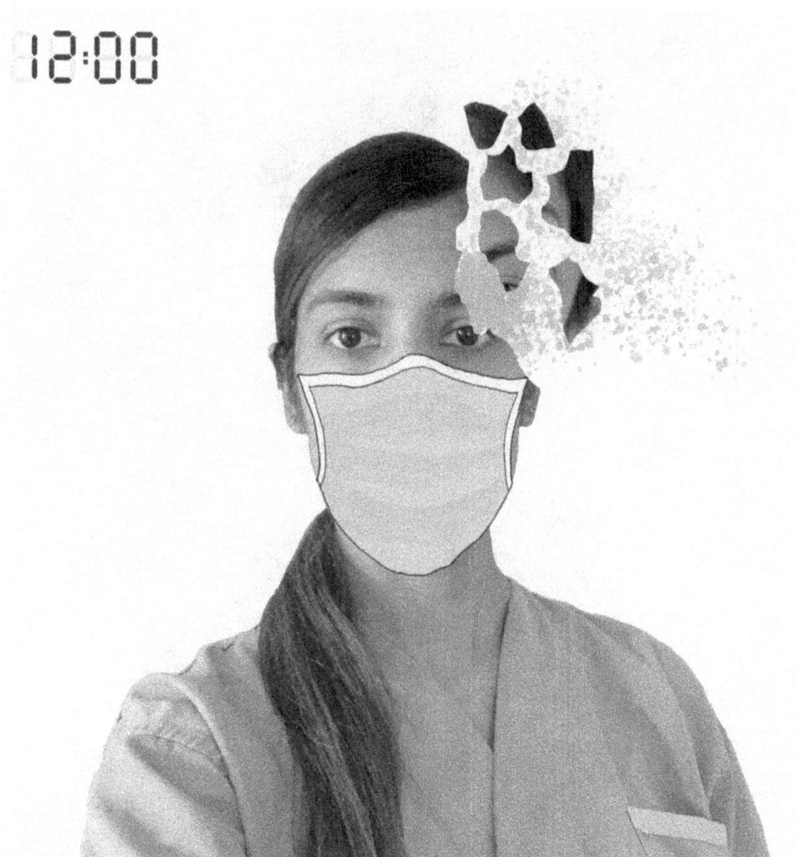
12:00

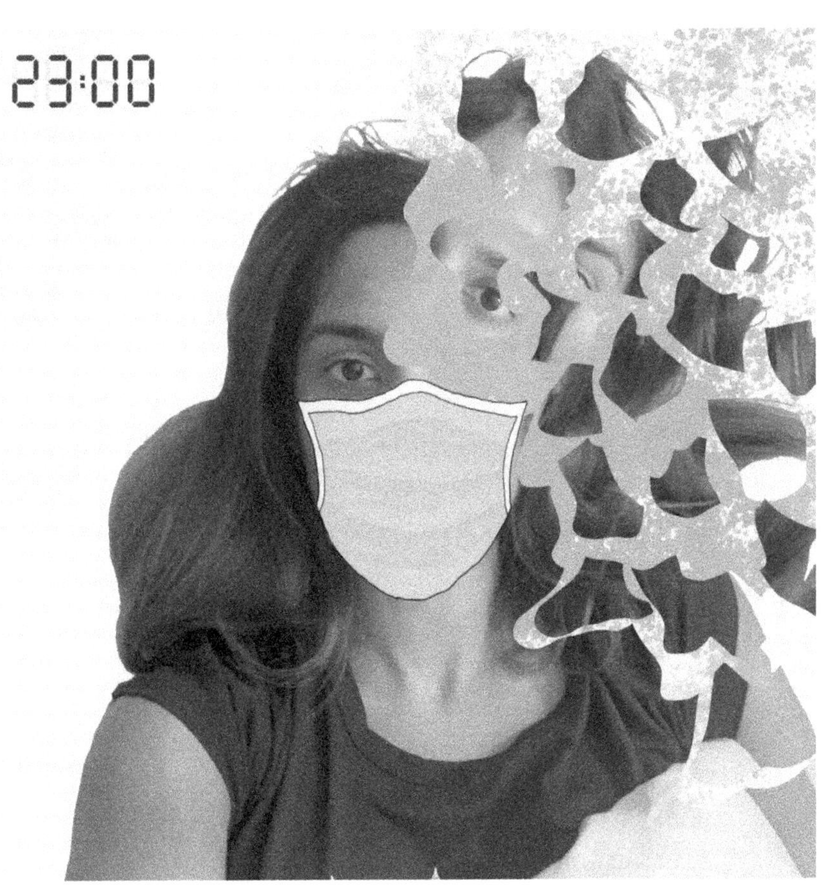
23:00

A Mask

MONICA KIDD

is two eyes & I see you
is an Aveda 821 Kashmir Brown kiss
is failing to hold a new father's beard
is appearing on the Prime Minister
is the tyranny of information
is a memo is a memo is a memo
is meant to sit on the nose
is a man sleeping under a bridge
is your screen time is up from last week
is a second wave, a third, an I've lost track
is what I meant when I said
is shouting in the wind
is teeth marks on my tongue
is a new wave of memes
is who can I trust
is a right-skewed curve
is breakfast for supper
is which side are you on
is my breath in my face
is a fashion accessory
is a brace of fuzzy dice

is falling like a petal
is a lonely night shift
is a string of beads
is my meandering horror
is flipping the bird
is contested
is a false negative
is empty shelves
is not a disguise
is gone
is gone
is gone

Facing the Unknown

Apprehensive, Overwhelmed, and Helpless

SHAN WANG

My name is Shan, I have recently obtained my college degree in nursing and will be pursuing a baccalaureate degree in nursing starting fall 2020. What follows this introduction is a collection of accumulated journal entries of a young woman who has volunteered to work in a nursing home located in Montreal, Quebec, during the pandemic. Lockdown in the province of Quebec has officially started on March 23. Two weeks later, I started working as a certified nursing assistant (CNA) in a nursing home qualified as a "hot zone," due to more than 60 per cent of the residents testing positive for COVID-19.

April 6, 2020

Here in Quebec, the working conditions in nursing homes are not ideal. The biggest issue lies in the ratio of the number of patients for one health-care provider. As an example, one CNA could be responsible for twenty to thirty patients and one nurse could be responsible for around one hundred patients (the number has climbed to around two hundred patients per nurse during the pandemic for a while due to major shortage of staff). Due to the unrealistic ratios, patient care is being neglected as health-care workers need to focus on prioritizing tasks and accomplishing as much as possible in the shortest amount of time possible.

Today was my first day of orientation as a temporary CNA. The shift started with a staff meeting. Management briefed us on how there are two confirmed COVID-19 cases on the floor and a recent death of a CNA who was still working a couple days ago. Management also announced that one floor will be completely converted to a COVID-19 floor, as will the recreational rooms be converted to COVID-19 rooms, to provide more rooms if needed. At the end of the meeting, management gave one box of surgical masks as well as five surgical masks with face shields attached to them to the nurse and asked her to lock everything up to prevent theft of the PPE. Worried, I asked how long the PPE she provided was supposed to last and if more is coming. She then instructed us to only use the PPE if we enter the two confirmed COVID-19 cases' rooms. The staff was hysterical; they realized they admitted one of the confirmed COVID-19 cases the day before with no PPE. They were afraid of potentially dying, especially since their colleague passed away a couple days prior.

Following and helping my orienteer with her tasks made me realize how difficult and demanding the job is, especially because she had around twenty-five patients to care for, while also having to do my orientation. Later that evening, the older CNAs regrouped to discuss resigning due to the risks of COVID-19. To this day, in this specific nursing home, the PPE worn when in contact with a confirmed COVID-19 patient are a surgical mask attached with a piece of plastic to act as an eye shield, a disposable jacket, and gloves. Social distancing, respiratory hygiene, and hand hygiene are the guidelines that we must follow in theory but are not respected in practice. The lack of PPE and the shortage of staff will lead to burned out and unprotected health-care providers. I came here to help but, unfortunately, I will have to resign and work elsewhere because

I do not feel safe in this specific work environment.

April 8, 2020

I was informed today that many units at the hospital have temporarily closed due to mandatory relocation of the hospital staff to the nursing homes. The ministerial decree makes it mandatory to work full time during the pandemic, and management took advantage of the situation to cancel any planned vacations of their employees. The PPE shortage is so bad the staff is limited to one surgical mask per day. Comparing ourselves to NYC, should we feel grateful we have disposable hospital gowns and don't need to use garbage bags as PPE? Isn't it the management's job to make sure their staff is well protected? Are we asking for too much? Some health-care workers are scared to work in an environment they do not feel safe in, so they decide to stop coming to work altogether. Management did not try to solve the issues and kept pushing their workers to work full time and overtime. Instead, management decided to hire new employees only to put them in the same working conditions.

People around me are worried about my involvement. I know it will be hard, especially because I am still a full-time student until the end of May, and working four days a week on top of that will be challenging. Since I am still living with my parents, I know I could put them at risk, but I will be taking all the precautions necessary to minimize the chances of potentially contaminating them. I can understand their concerns, but I just can't sit here and watch people die, so I made a decision and I'm holding myself accountable for my decision. After all, I decided on a career in health care because I wanted to take care of people and save as many lives as I possibly can. The government and the general public are calling us guardian angels and heroes. I find it flattering, but not helpful. I may be only speaking for myself, but all I ask for in exchange of putting myself and my colleagues at risk is proper PPE for all and for the general public to stay home and follow the guidelines.

April 9, 2020

I went out to do my groceries today. I avoid going as much as possible, but my supplies are running low, leaving me with no choice. I witnessed people in hysteria, panic-buying hand sanitizer, disinfectant wipes, masks, gloves, anything that would provide them some sense of security. I get it, people are scared because coronavirus is a new virus that can potentially be deadly, so they end up sheltering themselves, being skeptical of what the government is saying to them. They end up cross-contaminating themselves and their belongings because they are not using gloves and masks properly or worse, they wear N95 masks thinking they would protect them from the environment even though they have not been fitted for them and health-care workers are desperately in need of them. Not educating themselves properly can lead to hysteria and dangerous behaviours. Hysterical humans don't think before they act; they seek to blame and get revenge on those who they believe are the cause of their troubles. As a Chinese Canadian person, I find it scary to walk in the streets, fearing that I might encounter a racist person who is using coronavirus as an excuse to commit hate crimes against Asian people (which has happened a couple of times here in Montreal).

April 15, 2020

There is a rise in the number of staff burning out, having to stay home, or, in worst cases, being admitted to hospitals because they have tested positive for COVID-19. This is causing major issues to the already existing shortage of health-care providers (mostly nurses and CNAs). The premier of Quebec is now asking medical specialists to willingly come in nursing homes to work as nurses and CNAs. Since medical specialists have temporarily stopped consultations with patients due to the pandemic, it seems like it is a viable option. There is ruckus on my floor; the CNAs are dissatisfied with this decision. They are complaining, saying how they do not trust medical specialists because they believe they are the ones who pay the least attention to the prevention of infections since "they walk around everywhere with their lab coats." The CNAs are also upset because they heard the medical specialists will be paid $211/hour to do the same job as them. I find these comments upsetting and unnecessary. At a time like this, it is more important than ever to be unified as a team to work towards saving as many lives as we possibly can.

I have floated to a new nursing home. The working conditions here are better as there is food provided for us, enough PPE for all, and better ratios. I am being told to minimize all contact with residents who have tested positive for COVID-19, to only enter their rooms to feed them once, and change them once. Many residents have passed away because of their loneliness (as they have dementia and cannot comprehend the situation), and not from COVID-19 complications. The residents are letting themselves slowly rot away by refusing food and water. I feel helpless as we try our best but cannot prevent the deaths from happening. I keep seeing bodies wrapped in plastic bags on stretchers leaving the nursing home in little vans. It feels like this pandemic will never end, and as this goes on, I am realizing just how fragile human beings are.

April 16, 2020

The Government of Quebec has officialized the early deployment of students in health care who were to graduate this semester. In my case, this means I will be able to work as a "Candidate of the Nursing Profession" earlier than expected. I look forward to doing nursing interventions and evaluations again, it has been so long.

April 17, 2020

I just witnessed a CNA forcing medication on a patient. It made me feel uncomfortable because, in theory, the person preparing the medication is the person giving the medication. Since the CNA was gowned in protective gear and the auxiliary nurse was not, the auxiliary nurse gave the medication to the CNA to save time from gowning herself. My other issue with this is that I don't believe in forcing anything onto patients, even if they are unfit to make decisions for themselves. Rules are being bent, the staff is using shortcuts to save time and providing care of lesser quality. It is upsetting, especially if we consider our interactions with the residents might very well be their last interaction with a human being before they pass away...

My nursing home is labelled as a "hot zone"; this means that most of the residents here tested positive for COVID-19. On my floor, about fifty out of sixty residents are COVID positive. So far, ten residents have passed away and many more have their state deteriorating.

April 23, 2020

Today, we were only two CNAs who showed up for the sixty residents. As we are both nursing students and new to the job, it was quite worrisome. Fortunately, our team leader nurse found us three more CNAs to help us. Normally, as the floor is divided in three wings, at least two CNAs are in each wing. There are two auxiliary nurses on the floor and one team leader nurse for one to two floors, depending on the number of nurses available. Management has provided daily visits from one psychologist and one social worker. They have asked me how I was doing. I told them I did not feel safe enough without an eye shield that covers up our mouth area because the residents have been coughing on our faces and I doubt the surgical masks can protect us from particles projected onto our face. They told me to trust management and that they won't send us to take care of patients if they didn't think it was safe enough. I have my doubts about management's intentions but maybe that is just me?

My team leader nurse offered me to accompany him for his round. Many patients are under 4L of oxygen (4L being the limit a nursing home can provide because we will need N95 above 5L and currently do not have N95 in our nursing home). Antibiotics and fluids are given to patients in palliative care. The fluids (administered by subcutaneous and not by intravenous) are to replace the food and liquids that they're refusing to take.

April 24, 2020

Two residents started to cry in front of me today. One of them asked me for help her because she was afraid of dying. I stayed longer with her in hopes to reassure her and raise her spirits. The other one is paraplegic and the only resident apt to make decisions on her own. She has specific requirements as to how things must be done and when things must be done. I can understand her wanting to stay in control of what she still has control over, but being rude with the staff by calling us incompetent, amongst many other things, makes it difficult to feel empathy for her.

I was lucky enough to have a macaroon and a chocolate square for dessert, courtesy of the nursing home's free meal. It boosted my morale and made me feel better. It is really the littlest things that matter.

April 25, 2020

Being a CNA, especially during the pandemic, is starting to take a toll on me. It is mentally and physically draining. We were four CNAs today; I had a wing of around twenty residents for myself and it was quite difficult. I was a bit late since I took the time to feed a dysphagic resident by making sure he swallowed every bite. I feel discouraged, exhausted, and am starting to count down on the days I have left before the end of my contract as a CNA. The Quebec government is thinking of changing the name of the nursing homes from "CHLSD" (Centre d'hébergement de soins de longue durée, long-term care facility) to "Maison pour aînés" (home for the elderly) to make it more appealing to work in nursing homes. The premier is also considering increasing the salary of CNAs to attract more people into the profession. It is a good start but there is still a lot left to do, as CNAs often get injured when moving patients, feeding patients, changing patients. One CNA came to me to complain about her knee problems, telling me that her family doctor refused to give her a sick leave as "CNAS are necessary."

My colleague asked me for help in changing one of his residents. When we came in, she was rigid, her eyes were open, her mouth was semi-open with a white substance coming out of her mouth. We had the reflex to check her pulse and watch her breathing. There was no radial pulse on both sides, no carotid pulse, and no breathing at all. Her buttocks and extremities were cyanotic. We tried to straighten her and close her eyes but she was already too rigid. We then notified our team leader nurse who notified the doctor, who confirmed the death.

April 27, 2020

I got tested because I had a sore throat, a headache, occasional coughs with expectorations, diarrhea, but no fever. I received my result; it is negative but the lady from the health office wants me to be tested again because I am still symptomatic. I should be back to work if I get a second negative.

April 30, 2020

Management has started to admit new patients in the nursing home, ones that have tested both positive and negative for COVID-19. They have installed half-doors to lock them inside their rooms to "protect them from wandering to other rooms." This is to avoid the COVID negative residents to be contaminated and the COVID positive to contaminate. The new residents spend most of their times at their doors, asking us to let them out. It is difficult to witness all of this as it feels like they're animals locked in cages. I can understand management needs to make decisions to keep the economy going but I am worried it is a bit too early for admissions as many residents are still COVID positive. I will soon be starting my job as a candidate of the nursing profession; I can only hope that things will improve for the nursing home, for Quebec, for our country and the world in general...

I have reached out to Protection Collective, "a mutual aid network of makers in the Greater Montreal area who spontaneously began to manufacture Personal Protective Equipment (PPE) in order to offset the shortages and distribution of PPE to hospitals and healthcare facilities on the frontlines of the COVID-19 pandemic." They have generously provided us face shields as our management refused to do so. I am so grateful to this day for their work, they filled in a gap that was supposed to be taken care of by our management.

The prime minister has decided on sending the Canadian army to help in our nursing homes. It will be under Operation LASER, but, unfortunately, I will not be fortunate enough to work with them as my contract here will end beforehand.

May 5, 2020

As my contract is getting close to an end, I reminisce on the circumstances in which I wrote these journal entries. I wrote either during my break at work or very late at night after my shift. I experienced emotional ups and downs. There are times I felt so overwhelmed; I felt like I was crying and screaming on the inside. At other times, I felt emotionally numb and could not feel anything. I have been more anxious than usual and have trouble sleeping. This pandemic will have terrible consequences on the mental health of front liners and the general public, for sure.

I have worked as a maintenance worker beforehand for a summer and now I just got a taste of how it is to work as a CNA. This experience has taught me so much and made me understand my colleagues better by getting to see things from their perspective. As it is a problem today, I hope we can break down the medical hierarchy and work better as a team from here onwards.

On Pandemic and Uselessness

JAIME LENET

Sometime in March, they told us that visitors would no longer be permitted at the hospital. My heart broke for the patients and their families—already at their lowest, they were about to learn what it meant to be lower.

- A young single mom, separated from her child, not dying fast enough to qualify for "compassionate" visits
- An elderly woman with dementia believing that the only explanation for her family members' absence was that they were all dead
- A father with a newly acquired brain injury with impacts that had yet been observed by the family being told that he would not be coming home

They told us it was in their best interest. Maybe it was. That is not how it felt.

• • •

By late April, the virus had caused multiple outbreaks in long-term care. They requested "volunteers" to break from their day jobs—their *professions*—in order to *deploy* to these facilities.

The language of *deployment* is curious. Deploy, from the French word *deployer*, means to use something or someone in an effective way, or to move soldiers or equipment to a place where they are needed. I wondered quite a lot about how I might be used "in an effective way." What might I have to offer given that I had exactly no experience providing direct physical care? I was certainly no expert on infection control protocols. I had worked in hospitals for several years but had never once stepped foot into an institutional residence. Was I a soldier in some battle I did not understand? If so, who was the enemy, and how on earth was I to fight them? Did they really want someone of my weak constitution?

I stepped forward anyway.

Partly I think I went out of morbid curiosity. Here we were in the middle of what I assumed would be the most significant historical event of my lifetime. I didn't want it to pass me by. Long-term care homes had become the breeding ground for the virus, and I suppose I wanted to see what it really was all about. Was it as horrendous as all those Italian hospital workers had warned? Was all this panic much ado about nothing? I wanted to have stories for the next generation, and deep down I suppose I wanted my name on the record. Maybe I did it just so I could write this piece.

As I debated the risks to myself and my family, the physical demands of the job, the drop of status from *professional* social worker to personal care aid, I thought about the workers for whom this debate was not available. No one ever asked them if they minded the imminent health risks of their underpaid jobs. No one applauded their *heroic* decision to care for society's most vulnerable. No one provided them with assurances of proper training and access to PPE. It's hard to ignore that my decision had a lot to do with virtue signalling. I seized the situation as an opportunity to demonstrate my credentials as an ally to the *workers*. I felt compelled to demonstrate that my white professional class privilege did not prevent me from joining them *in the trenches*. Incidentally, these privileges did guarantee that I would be paid twice as much.

• • •

In early May I had my first shift on a locked unit for residents with dementia. Declining cognition was not new to me. A significant proportion of my usual clientele experience some form of cognitive impairment. But working with a physically unwell patient who is sometimes confused is worlds away from the institutional residence of two dozen individuals who can no longer make sense of their whereabouts or histories. Almost immediately after entering their space, the emotional labour of ignoring their losses quickly became exhausting.

Like clockwork every afternoon, for the past four years, one of the residents asks anyone she can find, "Where am I? When did I get here? What is this place? Where is my sister?" She is always surprised by the responses. Three days into this routine and I was fatigued by its fruitlessness.

Another resident—physically active and strong—walks circles around the unit non-stop hour after hour, day after day. He strings words together that have no collective meaning, but which carry a questioning tone to which no answer is satisfactory. They warned me not to let him stand too close. He hits.

To contain the virus, residents were ordered to stay in their rooms and to physically distance themselves from one another. Meals were to be eaten at bedside, and recreational materials were removed to discourage gatherings. Gone were the puzzles and art supplies, the dolls, and the board games. Gone was the fresh air and the visits from family. Remaining was the television playing a non-stop stream of pandemic news. Remaining were an endless number of hours passing by in slow motion on repeat.

Those whose minds were already failing found themselves in an oppressively unstimulating environment. I myself was confused about how I ended up there.

They resisted though. This social experiment held no allure to them. They went into each other's rooms. They ate off each other's plates. They hugged and kissed, and they held hands as they walked through the halls. One woman walked around with her arms constantly outstretched, reaching to experience the tactile sensation of absolutely every surface in the place. Had the virus made its way to this floor, there would surely have been little way to contain it. Then again, at least the puzzles couldn't be blamed.

• • •

Later, I was sent to another unit where the hallway was divided by one of those plastic walls you see in dystopian sci-fi movies (*Pandemic* maybe?). On one side were the residents who had tested positive, on my side were the ten who had not. I was assured of my safety and encouraged to follow the example of the personal support worker (PSW) assigned to work with me.

The woman I worked with that evening took me under her wing. She knew all the residents' habits and how they took their tea. She helped me feel useful by getting me to restock supplies, take meal orders, and assist with care. She was kind to the residents but also firm. If they didn't want to eat, she insisted. If they didn't want their brief changed, she did it anyway. She comforted me and told me, "That time, it wasn't so bad" when I was horrified by the resident who screamed and cried out for her mother the entire time that we washed her. She told me when to change my gloves and gown and when it was okay not to. She made sure I properly washed my hands, wrists, and arms before going on break.

That was Wednesday.

When I returned on Saturday, two of the residents had been moved to the "positive" side of the plastic wall and two more were on their way. By the end of that week, only four of the original ten remained and at least two had died. I had taken their meal orders on Wednesday and now they were dead. I don't know if the others recovered. But I checked the obituaries regularly.

I wondered when their infections occurred and if I might have been implicated. Had I changed my gloves often enough? Did I carry the virus on my sleeve from one room to another? Could it have been on my visor?

I was able to distance myself from these questions because the care of residents was not ultimately my responsibility. The PSWs I worked with—every single one racialized, all of them born outside of Canada—bore the full weight of responsibility and potential culpability. At the same time, they seemed to be given little to no input into how the residence was managed. Well before the pandemic brought their efforts into the spotlight, PSWs sorted through countless ethical dilemmas and emotional ordeals that media outlets could never seem to capture.

During my very short *deployment* in long-term care, I witnessed these *low-skilled workers* figured out what to do with a woman who refused to pull down her dress and a man who tried to hit them when they suggested he go to bed. I watched them decide if it was better to cause pain by repositioning a resident or to allow pressure sores to develop by leaving her alone. I relied on them to advise me on whether it was better to force fluids into a resident, or to risk their dehydration. For poverty wages, PSWs live with the weight of these decisions while their bodies are slammed with the physical consequences of providing care. In the pandemic, they also had to confront the possibility that they could be responsible for infecting a resident, and that their workplace could be responsible for infecting them.

• • •

When they asked us to stay on longer and to continue "helping," my commitment to the cause evaporated. I no longer wanted to bear witness to the desperate boredom of the residents, the heaviness of dignity lost, or the profanity of cheap labour being used to carry out some of the health system's most socially and ethically complex tasks.

I suppose I was disappointed. My *deployment* hadn't felt as though I had been used "in an effective way." It really only served to remind of my weaknesses.

Embracing the self-indulgence of my privilege, I went back to my hospital job where visitors were still prohibited, and I wondered at the violence of trusting a system to care for the people we love.

Pandemic

JORDAN PELC

Yes
I am a doctor
Saver of lives
Winner of awards for medical education
I've never failed an exam in my life

I have read the New England Journal of Medicine
And I am calling a meeting
I am calling a really big meeting
You should see the email I'm about to send

I am going to find my microscope
and use it
Engage in hand hygiene
like it's nobody's business
I'm going to fight this thing with science
With science
I'm going to hold the science in my hand
and fight

Prescription for Water

JIAMENG XU

When every door in society closed
I started telephoning strangers
We cannot get sick from listening
We cannot get sick from speaking into a machine
A woman in a lone room answers me
She thinks I am calling from her sister's care home.
Has her sister received a drink of water?
She asks me over and over
She worries because her sister is afraid to ask
There are people crying for help all around her
She does not want to become a burden.

When I was six years old
I carried a cup of water to my teacher
I held it beneath a metal tap
Liquid rose between my hands
Cold, heavy, and sure
She took the cup from my hands
Unburdening me of its weight

I did not know then what it meant to deal in burdens
Only tentative, unspoken gestures
Thirst, and coolness on my own lips
As I saw her drink.

It took me twenty years to learn
A drink of water is not a simple thing.
Somewhere in this city, beyond her sister's gaze
A woman is waiting
I do not know how much longer she must attend
In silence to the memory of water.
My own hands are empty
There is nothing to hold.

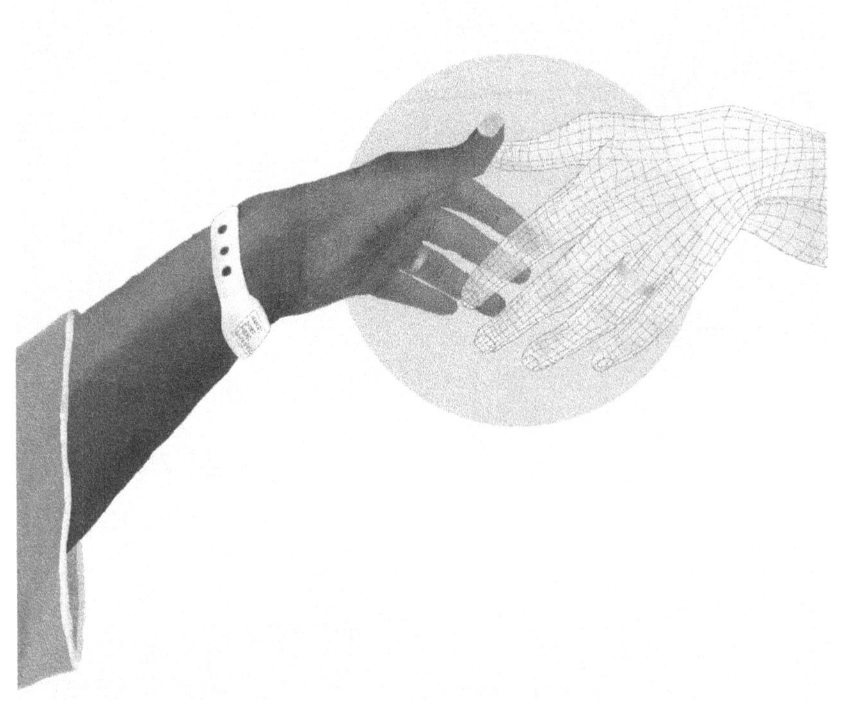

Palliative Care by Tharshika Thangarasa.
(First published as *Virtual Visitor* in the Spring 2021 issue of *Intima: A Journal of Narrative Medicine*.)

My So-Called COVID Life

JENNIFER MOORE

The details of my new patient consult appear in my pager in standard medical shorthand. I scan quickly through seemingly inconsequential details to find what is most relevant to me, the location of the patient. As a palliative medicine consultant, I see patients throughout the hospital, as suffering and dying are not relegated to one location. But like in real estate, in my job, location matters. If a patient is in a familiar unit, with familiar and collegial staff, I know my job will be easier. Better yet, if the staff is friendly, my experience will be more enjoyable.

Before the pandemic, I would be delighted to be asked to see a patient on the D4 ward. The D4 ward is a smaller ward in the hospital, with nurses and allied staff I especially enjoy working with. I looked forward to the heavy utilitarian doors opening inward and walking through to the sleek hospital unit with its tidy nursing station nestled in the centre. The renovation done last year made the unit even more pleasant. The fresh paint and lighting made a pleasant space even cleaner and brighter, with practical, comfortable workstations. No fighting for a place to sit with a computer as on other wards.

Though to be honest, I enjoy being most places in the hospital, as I truly feel comfortable here. For most people outside of medicine, the hospital may be a scary, horrible place. A place where bad things happen. But my most formative years occurred in hospitals and I love it here. Correction. Loved it here. In the months since the COVID pandemic began the hospital has come to feel eerie and strange. My second home is no longer a familiar place, no longer my sanctuary. And as the D4 ward is now designated as the hospital's main COVID ward, this pleasant space is no longer happy. Today, in my pandemic life, I stand outside D4 and activate the automated door with my ID badge. The doors open inward, just the same as they always did, but this time sounding like the opening of Darth Vader's ship as he exits to walk onto the Death Star. I enter the ward and the scene inside is equally cinematic, with nurses and doctors dressed in gowns, masks, and face shields. I search amongst these apparent space inhabitants for collegial faces, but masks blunt all identity. I can discern no familiarity in their faces. They could all be smiling in recognition at me, but I would never know.

I move cautiously towards the centre nursing station, careful to maintain two metres of distance as I thread my way through a team of nurses. I pause in front of a computer. This is a COVID unit, is it OK to touch the computer? Should I be wearing gloves? This worry hasn't occurred to me when accessing the computers on other hospital units. I glance to see if anyone else is typing on a computer and, if so, whether hands are gloved or not. As I scan the area I notice a box of gloves. I temporarily feel relief that the glove supply seems plentiful, but that joy is dampened by the sight of a box of masks which sits completely empty. While we have been reassured that our hospital has a good supply of masks, the sight of an empty box produces concern.

Our hospital has instituted a policy of distributing two masks to each employee daily. Each morning as I enter the building, I receive my masks in a brown paper bag, the same type of bag that I brought my lunch to school in as a child. I collect my masks from the station near the hospital entrance and clutch the bag greedily as I hurry to my office to change into hospital scrubs. I use my masks sparingly. Having one or two extra masks in my office soothes me but also can make me feel stingy, especially when I see an empty box on the ward. Yesterday a patient on the oncology ward tearfully told me how scared she was to be in the hospital. She had lost the paper mask she had brought with her when she was in the ambulance en route. She felt vulnerable without it. I returned with one of my spare masks in its brown paper bag and quietly gave it to her. Even though I gave her one from my own supply I felt guilty. Our eyes darted around furtively before the exchange to ensure no one saw us. Like a secret drug deal. Her eyes teared with gratitude and I felt good. Now as I see the shrinking supply of masks on the COVID ward my eyes tear up with worry for my colleagues and I feel anxious. Was I wrong to give a mask to a frightened patient? It wasn't an N95 mask, I rationalized. But worry nags me regarding my choice.

As I gather information from the patient's computerized chart, I glance up at the electronic monitor listing patients' names and room numbers on the ward. There is a new icon next to the room numbers, either an orange question mark or a red circle. The orange denotes a patient whose COVID test results are still pending; the red circle indicates a patient who is COVID positive. My patient has neither icon, as his COVID test was negative. I already knew this, but seeing neither colour next to his name still brings comfort. The relief in this information is temporary, as I watch an orange question mark suddenly disappear to be replaced with a red circle. I feel almost as if I am watching the virus replicate with the growing proportion of red dominating orange. I decide to refocus and go to see my patient. I struggle to place my face shield over my hair covering and mask. After interviewing and examining the patient, I exit his room, remove my gloves and sanitize my hands. As I rub hand sanitizer into my hands, I glance down at the ring finger of my left hand. Jewellery is now prohibited in the hospital so I have not worn my wedding ring in weeks. My hand still feels naked. While the computers in the nursing station remain unoccupied, I choose to leave the ward to return to my office to chart. This is a new habit for me. Previously I would have enjoyed the company of colleagues as I charted. I hate sitting in my office alone, but find myself doing that more and more.

I walk back to my office through empty hallways. The visitor restriction policy for hospitals has left the patients lonely and the halls feeling hollow. A few staff members pass me in the hall. Before the pandemic I enjoyed seeing familiar faces of staff I otherwise didn't know. We would exchange a smile as we passed each other. I miss smiles. Now we pass each other in masks with unknown expressions underneath. In my first few days back, I tried greeting people with muffled hellos, but was never quite sure if anyone actually heard me. Then there were a few days when I tried raising my eyebrows in greeting, but that began to feel creepy. Plus, the action gave me a headache. I considered trying out what I only can describe as the "dude nod," that silent, half raise of the head or chin, most commonly seen as an exchange of acknowledgement between young men. I contemplated doing that to replace my smile of hello, but stopped short, worrying that I looked more like I had some neurologic tic, rather than was attempting a greeting.

I had been in the US when the pandemic was declared, forcing me to quarantine at home for two weeks prior to returning to work. On my first day back, I felt nervous and out of place. My colleagues had a two-week head start on adjusting to the new life inside the hospital walls and seemed unaware to my uncertainties. That morning when I exited the parking lot, I walked to my usual entrance to the hospital only to find the doors sealed closed. I wandered to the next entrance and was relieved to enter the doors the same time as a friend. The guard at the entrance startled as I attempted to walk straight through and my friend quickly instructed me on the new procedure. "Wait, stop. Show your badge and then get some hand sanitizer.

Wash your hands in front of the guard to show that your hands are clean." I had always joked with my children that at my work there were "hand washing police," but this was the closest to that reality I had ever encountered. My friend then steered me to the mask distribution area to collect my two face masks. With those tasks complete, I found my way to my office, anxious to connect with my co-workers. Co-workers I had not seen in two weeks. But I found no one socializing in the halls. Office doors were closed with inhabitants inside practising social distancing. Our morning team meeting with colleagues sitting around a table is replaced with a Zoom meeting. I can hear the echoes in the hallway when my teammates speak, but they still feel far away. The frequent freezing on Zoom only heightens isolation.

On that first day back, I quickly began using hospital-supplied iPads to FaceTime with family members when I was at patients' bedsides. The challenges and inadequacies of this intervention quickly became apparent. For some families, seeing their loved ones sicker or newly confused on FaceTime brought no comfort, only accentuating distress. One family member found FaceTiming with his loved one particularly distressing. He begged me on the phone to allow him to come in and be by the patient's bedside. A request I was desperate to grant but had no authority to. In another room I witnessed an emotional FaceTime between a patient and the patient's adult child. They both were weeping while the patient kissed her fingertips and touched the child's face on the screen. At the end of the call I took the hospital iPad encased inside a plastic bag from the patient's hands. The patient dried her tears and turned to me and said, "Well, that was nice. But now you are going to walk out that door and I am again going to be all alone." The loneliness in the room was palpable and I found myself at a loss for words to respond. Each patient visit brought fresh, raw emotions. At the end of the day, I felt emotionally dehydrated. When I left that day, I walked towards my usual exit only to find the door sealed and needed to backtrack to the accessible exit.

Now I lock my office to change out of my scrubs. I carefully place the scrubs into a cloth bag that is washer safe and can be tossed in at home along with my clothes. My head covering follows the scrubs into the bag. The cloth bag gets tied and placed into a second bag, all a ritual I now perform daily in an attempt to minimize any rogue virus invading my home. I change my shoes and tuck my newly baptized "hospital shoes" under my desk. As a working mom of three, laundry has always been my nemesis. But with my new COVID life, laundry has multiplied as I wear three outfits in a day. My hospital scrubs, clothes I change into to wear home from work, and clothes I change into after a shower at home. The increase in volume of laundry is further complicated by the need to keep my laundry separate from the rest of the family's laundry. I lock my office door and abruptly stop myself as I gaze down at my ID. Once again I forgot to sanitize my badge, a recommended essential step for infectious disease prevention. I unlock my office and grab a disinfectant wipe. After sanitizing my ID badge, I lock my office and head towards the accessible exit.

My walk to the parking garage allows me an opportunity to revel in a COVID silver lining—the parking lot is emptier than it was prior to the pandemic. There is a sense of smug satisfaction that I have a parking spot on the fourth floor of the garage rather than my standard sixth floor location. Fewer stairs to climb at the end of the day. I am exhausted and therefore grateful. I drive out of the garage towards the exit. As I turn onto the city road, I am still surprised at the emptiness of the streets. While little traffic on the roads is another small COVID silver lining, it feels aching and empty to see the world devoid of people and cars. A colleague from a different hospital calls me on my way home. I am eager to talk, to connect. We both are struggling with our new normal. Our exchange teeters from distress to raucous laughter as we review our day. None of our conversation captures the deeper currents of our experiences, but the laughter heals us. At one point I pull over as I am laughing hard. I tell her about the time I was in a patient's room with my face shield slowly creeping up my face. The strap of the shield had caught on my ponytail. I didn't want to touch my face while in the room and silently willed my hair follicles to keep the shield from rocketing off my head. At the end of another visit my glasses and face shield were both so fogged up not only could I not see the patient, but I struggled to navigate exiting. I wonder how disconcerting it must be for patients to see physicians floundering. We commiserate and laugh. For a few moments I forget. I forget we are in a pandemic, the streets are ghostly, and that I may be carrying a deadly virus on my hair, clothes, and person. I pull into my driveway lost in the momentary reprieve.

My husband and I have carefully planned how I re-enter the home from work to prevent viral exposure. The plan is important to me, as I fear exposing my family. We are fortunate enough to have a basement with a shower, accessible from a side door of the house. I enter and bypass my family and main living area. Once in the basement shower, I complete a ritualistic decontamination process. My children will often see me as I sneak in the side door, but back away cautiously, only happy to connect once I have showered. Our dog often bounds toward the side door, tail wagging and happy to see me. My children pull him back, terrified he will be infected.

Today is different. The phone call with my friend has cheered me and caused me to forget. Even though we are commiserating on this new strange life, I forget the pandemic and cautious re-entry. I forget I am a viral threat to the inhabitants of my home. I exit the car and bound up my front stairs while saying my goodbye. My phone call ends and I enter the front door of my house with cheer, eager to see my family. As I step into the house pandemonium ensues. "What are you doing?" screams a voice, followed by "Why is mom coming through the front door?" The dog bounds up towards me, happy to see me, but the rest of my family backs away in fear. I am told, not asked, to stick to procedure and go back out. The request is simple and reasonable. But the emotion of the message stings. I feel like a pariah. A pariah whose family is telling her to get out.

I step out the front door and stand a moment on the porch. I have heard so many colleagues speak of their fear of infecting their families. I, myself, worry about infecting my family. But in this moment, I feel a sting of rejection. Intellectually I know it is not a rejection, but the feeling permeates me. The magnitude of being unable to enter my home through the front door saddens me, dissolving the feelings of goodness and connection I had just received. I take a deep breath to try to shake of the sadness and turn to walk down the front steps. My eyes catch sight of a child's drawing in the window of a neighbour's house. A rainbow, a sign of hope. Underneath the rainbow the childish scrawl, "We are all in this together." I repeat the phrase in my head, "We are all in this together." I wonder then why, in this moment, do I feel so alone?

Pulling Strings

MONIKA DUTT

We had finished a strange COVID-19 pandemic summer, floating through a new kind of world, seeing few people, moving in the tiniest geographic area. Cape Breton like I'd never seen it, without the beach gatherings, musical celebrations, grand tourist events; but still Cape Breton. Somehow.

Cough. Cough.

My heart sank as I listened to my nine-year-old son Kail coughing in his bedroom next door. This was the first sign of illness since being back at school. At least my child was in school, unlike many parts of the country where kids had been in and out of in-person classes, mainly out.

"Are you really sick?" I asked him, somewhat accusingly. I stood at the doorway, a good three metres away.

"I'm sorry, Ma," he said, wiping his blanket across his runny nose.

"Oh *mishti*, I'm sorry. I know you're sick." I paused. "And you're going to get a COVID test."

"COVID?" His eyes widened. "Do I have COVID?" His tiny voice grew louder.

“No. I’m sure you don’t.” I spoke with the confidence of a public health physician who knew that locally, at the time, there had been few people diagnosed with COVID-19, while hiding the doubt of a mother worried that their child could be *the one*. I backed away another step.

“Here’s a mask to wear in the house.”

Kail’s sickness made me obsessively diligent. I was *not* going to get sick. We were going to be the best mask-wearers, hand-washers, and distance-keepers ever. I had been working virtually from home as a medical officer of health for Newfoundland and Labrador since the pandemic had started, so my head was full with ways to beat this virus. I even implemented infection prevention protocols in the house.

“You take the upstairs bathroom. I’ll take the downstairs. You can’t use my bathroom.”

“Okay, Ma,” he said, his brown eyes wide and obedient.

“And this is your towel. And we can’t share food or drinks.”

“Okay, Ma.”

I continued in the car. “You sit in the back, diagonal from me.” Once positioned, I opened all the windows. It was a bit chilly, but the masks helped to keep our faces warm. Sort of. “Kail! Don’t touch your mask!” He looked at me, embarrassed, and quietly placed his hands in his lap. I gave him sanitizer and he dutifully rubbed his hands, just like they had taught him on the first day back at school. Beside him was an iPad playing his favourite Percy Jackson book, a fantasy adventure based on Greek mythology featuring a boy who fights both with and for gods and goddesses pulling the strings of humanity.

When it was time to have the swab inserted in his nose, he leaned his head back. His bouncy, curly hair surrounded his smooth, deep brown face.

“You may have some tears,” the nurse warned him, then stuck the long swab in. He yelped involuntarily, but remained still, a tear easing down his check.

“You didn’t tell me it would hurt like that,” he said accusingly when we walked out. He reached for my hand. I held it, briefly. Then I re-sanitized back in the car.

• • •

Overnight the provincial lab sent new results for people who were COVID-19 positive and my mind swam from the first second of waking, the pandemic an extension of my being. These alerts beckoned more than any social media notification. Each one held a story. A child who had been in school, played with sports teams, attended a birthday party; a worker who had to spend more time in a mine in Alberta than with his family; an infectious staff member working in a long-term care home.

There had been surges in other parts of Newfoundland and Labrador, but then it happened in the region I was responsible for. The alerts were relentless:

10 new positive results.
14 new positive results.
40 new positive results.

Much of the rest of the country would scoff at the small numbers. But we were in Atlantic Canada, the bastion of near COVID-zero, where schools had been open most of the year and live music was starting up as summer eased around the corner. I didn't want to be the one who shattered the mostly flat line on the graph.

Public health staff were brittle; I could see the exhaustion on the nurses' faces. "I'll work tomorrow if I need to. But this has been hard," one said, her voice wavering. "I'm alone with my kids, I don't have childcare, and I don't know if I can do this."

The nurses were an interface with human impact. They delivered the shocking news of a positive result, dealt with tears, disbelief, sometimes anger, then tried to move on to elicit helpful information. They absorbed the anguish of the woman who had transmitted the infection to her ninety-four-year-old grandparent, comforted the child ostracized because she was the one who had unknowingly brought the infection to school.

As a public health physician, I gave medical advice on management and strategy. There was sometimes a rush to that, in imbibing the constantly evolving evidence from a fountain then applying it, the intellectual rigour of hashing through approaches with other medical officers of health. I was supposed to be an expert on so many aspects of this virus, and I hungrily read, watched, and learned all I could, just to realize I needed to update my knowledge the next day.

However, learning was a luxury between questions and meetings; the phone didn't stop ringing, the emails were incessant.

> He's positive, and he's a lobster fisherman who works on his own. He's not supposed to leave his house, but he'll lose his catch and significant income if he doesn't go out on his boat. What should he do?

> She carried a cabinet with her father, indoors, no mask, less than two metres, while she was infectious. Is her father at risk?

> All shelter residents and staff have been moved to a hotel due to the exposure to someone who was positive. They need the staff who were exposed to keep working so they can function. How do we do that?

I imagined a COVID-19 cloud, darting in, out, and around us. Making decisions for people I'd never met, I recognized that my recommendations impacted whether people could go back to work, visit a dying parent, get sick, or even die. At other times I knew that little I did mattered considering that people still lacked basics like safe housing and paid sick days, and the workers most at risk were undervalued by those with the most power. When I saw patients in my family medicine clinic, I saw close-up how devastated peoples' lives were by pandemic measures that worsened the unjust situations they had already been put in. I knew I was part of the system that imposed measures that often helped and also often harmed.

The emergence of self-created public health "experts," and the way the media relied on them, added unexpected frustrations. People with little public health background but good skills at sharing sound bites became media sensations. Skepticism towards information coming from public health physicians was encouraged by routinely introducing commentators from other specialties as being "independent" on their newscasts. Media seemed to relish critiques from people who would not be held accountable for the policy recommendations they tossed out in the way that medical officers of health would be. Some MOHs were threatened, others had protests in front of their houses.

Social media was another troubling force. Comments towards public health alternated between revering, questioning, and sometimes intimidating. Scrolling through Twitter late one night I read this description by a physician colleague about public health physicians: "Well meaning...not independent—political priorities can often trump medical ones...limited job market, often don't have a clinical practice they can fall back on..." Policy critiques I could deal with, that was the nature of working in a cloud of constantly evolving evidence. It was the undermining and personal attacks that were hurtful, yet impossible to ignore.

• • •

"Ma?" I heard his small voice from the living room. I was in my office, distracted. The metaphorical COVID wave felt real, a wall of water moving inexorably towards me, while an under-resourced public health team tried desperately to build a dam.

"What Kail?"

"My throat hurts."

I walked out of my office to look over the railing at him on the couch.

"How about writing in your journal? Talk about how you feel."

"Okay," he responded listlessly. I returned to my office.

Later that night I was in the kitchen. Kail had gotten ready for bed and we had called out our goodnights, snuggles postponed until he recovered. I saw his notebook on the table. Taking unjust motherly liberty, I opened today's page.

I am sick. I hate being sick. I can't do anything
And the worst part is that I can't even hug Ma.

I ran up the stairs to Kail's room. He was curled up under his blanket on one side of his bed, his four stuffies tucked in on the other side. Artemis, Athena, Poseidon, and Zeus, after his four favourite Greek gods and goddess.

I closed my eyes and leaned my cheek onto his back. Over his shoulder I could see his stuffies. They looked back at me. Was it with judgement or approval?

"Ma?" he asked, half-asleep. I crawled into the bed beside him. "But Ma, I'm sick!" he protested.

"I know," I said, wondering if I was providing healing energy or tempting fate.

Disembodied

An Examination of the Examination in a Pandemic

LIAM DURCAN

It happened about six weeks after our apps, followed in short order by the World Health Organization, told us it was coming. Once the lockdowns had been announced, the sports leagues suspended and the streets emptied, once we'd been introduced to our previously anonymous chief health officers from behind their banks of microphones and our commutes to work had resolved into an oddly unsatisfying series of uncontested left turns, I finally accepted that my patients had disappeared.

A full day's schedule of clinic patients had accepted the newly available option of a telemedicine visit. No one would be coming to the clinic. In a time of sudden and widespread upheaval, heightened risk and anxiety, this disappearance felt reasonable. Even rational. The thought of working from home and fighting for bandwidth with my Zoom-schooled teenage children was incentive enough for me to continue going to the clinic every day and making all my videoconference or telephone calls from the same chair in the same office. More practically, keeping a regular daily schedule in the clinic allowed me to be present should anyone need to be seen in person. Eventually, I was able to admit that going in every day was probably more of a mental health strategy, a way of dealing with (admittedly through sublimation) something that troubled me. I sat in the same chair, behind the same desk and stared at the same computer monitor during these interactions. Another chair, now empty, sat on the other side of the desk. I wore my lab coat and thought about my ergonomic shortcomings more and began what would become a slow but certain descent into a particular despair about my work.

Despair, was, of course, the dominant mood. A novel, communicable, and potentially lethal illness for which there was no clear treatment meant simultaneous medical, social, and economic crises. In a situation where people die or jobs and houses are lost or anxiety becomes the ever-inflating central currency of discourse, I understand that having one's patients disappear is not a comparable grievance but it was the change in my life that I found the most perplexing.

The patients I did see, usually during my weeks of hospital service doing general neurology consults or as a physician member of the stroke service, *were* sick, either ill enough with COVID to be admitted or so ill with a non-COVID illness that the spectre of going to a hospital filled with COVID patients was the lesser of two evils. For these patients, we were introduced to the rituals of our new medical lives, the categorization of risks and their mitigation through distance and layers and hygiene. Every act was an elaboration of distance, all interactions with patients were mediated through new barriers. Mask and visor, gown and glove. We donned our gear and went about our business suited up like this. Patient histories were degraded into to the broadest of dialogue and gesture, like some amateur theatre production featuring representatives from rival space programs. The physical exam suffered even more, streamlining itself in that way that inconvenience and anxiety conspire to accomplish.

The physical exam is an important act for any doctor, but for neurologists, it has always carried a special meaning. It's our thing. We measure the size of the pupils. We scan the skin of bare-limbed patients looking for a trace quiver that could be the first fasciculations of Lou Gehrig's disease. We count the blinks per minute of the patient with a change in handwriting to determine if signs of Parkinson's disease are present. From the moment Wilhelm Erb and Carl Westphal described the stretch reflex in 1875, neurologists recognized the value of the exam, an objective assessment in a universe of sometimes unfathomable patient symptoms. In 1896 Joseph Babinski was the first to describe the extensor plantar responses in his search for signs that would help differentiate organic neurological dysfunction from functional presentations that Jean-Martin Charcot, his mentor, felt were best evaluated by history and close observation. In the thirty years that followed these first steps, neurologists—a generation of intrepid clinicians in France, Germany, and England—created and codified an increasingly elaborate examination.

To neurologists, the justification for the demands of the examination lay in the complexity of the organ system whose truths it was charged with revealing. To more than a few non-neurologists, the exam was unnecessarily—and purposefully—arcane and seemed more of a compensatory facade for what they felt was the specialty's historical inability to do anything more than localize a problem. But neurologists were undaunted.

I was discovering that the examination was more than just a checklist or a simple addendum to the patient's narrative understanding of their experience. I discovered, later in the summer when infection rates declined and patients finally agreed to appear for an exam after a first telephone contact, that I had a diminished recollection of a patient if I had not physically examined them, as though I needed to incorporate the semantic meanings of their illness into the more procedural memory of an exam. The exam, I now understood was a physical representation of their state that I needed to integrate to properly to form a concept not just of their problem, but of the patient themselves. The first months of the pandemic were an exercise in trying to find ways to understand my patients without this key part of my interaction with them.

I worked hard to optimize my practice for those patients who wouldn't come into the office. I studied technique, watched webinars on communication strategies, and created scripts if I found a phrase or line of questioning that worked particularly well. I like to think I cultivated a warm tone and became a better listener, and I think that many of my patients were gratified that we could safely keep a therapeutic relationship alive under the trying circumstances of a pandemic. I like to think, sitting at one end of a conversation, that I *witnessed*. My patients seemed happy.

I was miserable.

I was waking up earlier and was losing my patience at home and while it was tempting to invoke COVID as the cause, the default for unhappiness, that seemed simplistic. I like my patients and find my work satisfying, but the thought of another day of phone calls, much less endless weeks of phone calls, saddened me. Despite my efforts to improve questioning to better understand the narrative basis of my patient's problem, to compensate for not having access to the physical aspects of their problem, the information I was getting in these conversations was insufficient. I was unsatisfied. I felt like someone systematically deprived of necessary information. Even patients seeking a new consultation were declining to come to the clinic and my sense that something vital was being missed, concealed by this new arrangement, was feeding a sense of panic.

I've looked after patients whose neurological deficits were best thought of as a loss of information input: the stroke victim who is left without vision, the person whose inflammatory nerve disorder has left them unable to sense the position of their limbs. Sometimes, in the wake of these deficits, other functions flourish—a heightened tactile ability develops or a sense of hearing becomes more acute in those who've become blind. Occasionally, the brain, deprived of input, simply creates its own experience: visual hallucinations are not infrequently experienced by the blind in the Charles Bonnet syndrome, and those who have lost sensation in a limb sometimes report an altered sense of the size of the limb. I had no such windfalls of insight or blossoming of technique, my skills as a communicator, as an interrogator on the phone remained resolutely unchanged and so my situation seemed instead like that of a person afflicted by a phantom limb, my response to a loss memorialized by a slow smoldering ache.

I've always been interested in the nature of the clinical interaction, how a patient's positive expectation could create an intangible benefit. I saw, as a medical student, that doctors who were genuinely friendly and reassuring, without being dismissive or patronizing, had patients who were not just more satisfied, but appeared to have better outcomes. It seemed as though there was something about certain doctors, or about the way they conducted themselves, that achieved more for their patients. Like anyone learning a craft, I tried to model my behaviour in clinical interactions after colleagues whose manner I found therapeutic, trying to mimic their equanimity, trying to summon their deep interest in the task at hand. Researchers in the neurobiological underpinnings of the placebo response, like the University of Turin's Fabrizio Benedetti, have looked at the psychosocial context of the clinical act and proposed that many of the same mechanisms underlying placebo response—expectation, classical conditioning—are at work when we encounter and examine a patient. My practice, in conscious and, I suspect, in unconscious ways, became a laboratory in adopting behaviours that attempted to maximize these intangible benefits. The way I positioned myself in the office, my tone of voice, and the manner in which I greeted patients in a crowded waiting room, the way I held a reflex hammer or the words I used as the patient stood to begin their departure, all these acts were honed in the direction of therapeutic benefit, because, if they are not, in what direction do they carry?

Part of that interaction, a huge part, I've come to understand, is what occurs during the physical examination. The exam, as internist and author Abraham Verghese points out, is a ritual with its specific setting and roles and symbolic tools. And as ritual, its power as a sociocultural apparatus is amplified, making it capable of creating significant positive or negative results (just as a placebo effect is possible, so too is the nocebo). Verghese, as though speaking to me in my empty office, goes further in his estimation of the importance of the examination, saying that the "human-to-human rituals in medicine benefit not only patients; they also help to relieve the dysphoria and disillusion existing in a medical system that is often technologically proficient but emotionally deficient" (Costanzo and Verghese 2018, 426).

Just reconsidering the exam in this way, as not just another investigative tool or mandated task but as a valued act with potential therapeutic benefit, is affirming, especially at a time when the patient interaction seems to compete in a zero-sum battle with other demands of care. The pandemic that emptied the examination rooms while maintaining a physician's responsibility for patients had not caused this as much as suddenly made this plain.

But attitudes about what goes on in a doctor-patient interaction are varied, and not all bear Verghese's affirming view. In Foucault's *Birth of the Clinic*, an analysis of the emergence of modern medicine, an alternate view of the examination is considered. Here, it is not seen as a potentially therapeutic tool, but exists as a strictly maintained manifestation of the power dynamic between doctor and patient. The physical examination is one of the ways—the most proximate, the most personalized—that clinical observation is generated and becomes a key element in the development of what Foucault coins "the medical gaze," all of which he argues marks a shift in which the perceptions of the doctor became more credible than those of the patient. In this way, the exam becomes a ritual of an entirely different sort to that described by Verghese. In reading

Foucault, any doctor's intentions, including mine, are called into question, and I can't help but be unsettled at the prospect that I may be bemoaning being deprived not of the possibility of helping or understanding, but of the opportunity to be proven right, of being able to fully exert my authority.

A resolution of these seemingly rival concepts may be found in notions of embodiment that originate outside of a neurological or medical framework. Anthropologists use the term *embodiment* as a way of describing experience as it is informed by factors such as gender, race, sexuality, or socioeconomic status, an exercise increasingly incorporated into medical curricula as a way to more fully serve patient needs. Costanzo and Verghese (2018) reference the work of Nora Jones, an anthropologist and associate professor of medicine at Temple University, who reconsiders the notion of patient interaction as a tripartite framework looking at the body as specimen (as seen by the clinician), as spectacle (an example of disease in popular culture), and as patient (the patient's understanding of their own body).

In this framework, Foucault's thesis informs but does not disqualify the concept of examination as a healing act, just as it reminds clinicians that their observations are not untouched by bias but always occur in a context that must be acknowledged.

I was thinking of all this during a recent elevator ride in the hospital during a week of consultations. When I attend the consultation service, I carry my doctor's bag. It's practical; a neurologist has tools they must carry to do their work. It is an object of many beautiful features even when emptied of tools—the heft and texture, the warmth of aged leather and the hinges upon which the bag opens, the handle—that is somehow organized into an object more beautiful than the sum of its parts. It is also, without doubt, the one thing about me that draws comments from complete strangers and passersby, be they patients, hospital visitors, or even staff. These exchanges may occur in a hallway or in a pod in the emergency room, but usually they take place in the silence and stillness of a half-empty elevator where, typically, the person next to me will point to the bag and, without exception, tell me that the sight of it pleases them. It gives them some sense of comfort. One such moment occurred in the last week. I held up the bag a little closer to the person with both hands, like it was a presentation object. She extended an index finger and touched its surface.

What I didn't tell her is that my doctor's bag was a gift, given to me in the earliest days of my career from my father-in-law who had died in hospital just weeks before this elevator ride, who did not die from the virus but whose last days were nonetheless marked by the new rituals of distance and isolation that have come to define medical experiences now. That memory, of my father-in-law in an ICU bed, a much-loved man dying in a diorama of Foucaultian prophecies, is now carried in the bag along with whatever reassurances it may provide to others. It is my bag to carry, its weight, its warnings and promises. I took a disposable cleaning wipe and rubbed the spot on the bag where the person had touched it and went about the rest of my day.

References

Costanzo, Cari, and Abraham Verghese. 2018. "The Physical Examination as Ritual: Social Sciences and Embodiment in the Context of the Physical Examination." *Medical Clinics of North America* 102 (3): 425–31. https://doi.org/10.1016/j.mcna.2017.12.004.

Foucault, Michel. (1973). 2003. *The Birth of the Clinic: An Archeology of Medical Perception.* Translated by A.M. Sheridan. New York: Routledge.

Jones, Nora L. 2011. "Embodied Ethics: From the Body as Specimen and Spectacle to the Body as Patient." In *A Companion to the Anthropology of the Body and Embodiment*, edited by Frances E. Mascia-Lees, 72–85. West Sussex: Blackwell Publishing.

Same But Different

DAVID GRATZER

I show my hospital photo ID, and he takes a quick look. He then asks me the screening questions about possible symptoms and recent travel. I quickly answer, trying not to be short with him, but eager to get to my office and start the day. He thanks me, and hands me a small sticker for my badge. I nod and walk past the other screeners, the new ritual of entering a hospital at a time of outbreak.

But the year isn't 2020, and I'm not an attending psychiatrist. It's 2003, and I'm in my third year of residency. SARS is burning in Toronto hospitals; COVID-19 lies far in the future.

So many things are similar if a bit different. Then as now, there is uncertainty. Rumours travel quickly. We all have opinions—how long the outbreak will last, where it will spread, etc.—but we know far less than we would like.

I tend to look forward, and not backwards. After the SARS left Toronto in the summer of 2003, I've rarely thought about it. But when COVID-19 was declared a pandemic, I've thought much about the *other* big outbreak, which affected twenty-six countries.

Two things strike me as different today, having worked through SARS so many years ago.

First, I'm different.

I was in my mid-twenties during SARS. I had been a doctor for under three years. Of course, I had never lived through an epidemic—or, frankly, thought much about one.

I remember feeling that SARS wasn't quite real.

While I didn't enjoy SARS, I greeted the virus like a new adventure. There were new policies and procedures and practices, daily puzzles to work on. There were new stories told—often third or fourth hand—about how people presented with the virus. I wasn't scared; I was intrigued.

I'm now at a different point in my life and my career. SARS struck just before my wedding; today, my wife and I live with our three children. I graduated from medical school two decades ago; the rescue fantasy is still there, but it's been tempered by time and experience.

And I see things differently with COVID. I'm curious—but my feelings are coloured by concern and, sometimes, dread.

And I worry. I worry about my patients and how they are coping, about their jobs, about their families. I remember working though the last recession (2009) in Scarborough, and remember how difficult it was for my working-poor patients, with the uncertainty and the angst. This could be worse.

I worry too about people I haven't met. Lying in bed at night, for example, I wonder if the suicide rate will go up. How many people will die indirectly from this virus? What can be done? Sometimes it's tough not to take my hospital job home with me. I serve on many committees, and we have spent months thinking through different scenarios, many of them hard. One stuck with me—if there are many deaths at College St. site, where would the bodies go? (There's no morgue.) I'm not sure why this scenario turned over in my mind, but it has, over and over.

And I also appreciate more.

I interact with many clinical and administrative teams. Though there have been moments of tension, I note how well people have worked together. In particular, I'm surprised by how well doctors are getting along. Grand rounds are well attended. People volunteer to help their colleagues out. Doctors text each other silly COVID-19 jokes. One of the drawbacks of working in a big hospital like the Centre for Addiction and Mental Health is that you can feel isolated; these days, I feel part of a vibrant medical community. And I appreciate all this.

Second, mental health care is different.

When SARS was declared an outbreak, I had just switched from an inpatient rotation to an outpatient one. For two days, I came to my office. For two days, I read emails, caught up on papers that I had wanted to read but hadn't, and talked with colleagues on the phone.

Clinically, I cancelled my outpatient appointments as the hospital was closed to all but inpatients and emergency department patients, but I didn't think much about it. I would reconnect with them sooner rather than later. I wasn't sure when, but I wasn't particularly concerned, either. Telepsychiatry was small in those days, the technology confined to a dedicated clinic that connected with clinics in remote communities. While I could talk to my patients by phone, there was no opportunity for televideo.

After a couple of days, I stopped coming to the hospital. After all, I could read emails from home.

Today, our outpatient services continue on. Through lockdowns, we have used digital platforms, and telepsychiatry has surged here (up 850 per cent from March to April 2020) and across North America (a *Psychiatric Services* paper surveyed twenty psychiatrists who are all using virtual visits; the majority hadn't used it before the pandemic) (Uscher-Pines et al. 2020).

When I speak to patients, I'm struck by how services have changed—a young woman who finds an app helpful; an older man who is now attending a virtual group; a young man who will start an e-therapy program in the coming weeks.

SARS shut down my clinical work; COVID has made me pivot.

And COVID has also made me think about SARS, about how we deal with such challenges, and—reassuringly—how they end. In a few years, I know, one of our energetic, young colleagues will be talking about their experiences during the great pandemic of 2020 (and 2021, 2022, and 2023).

Reference

Uscher-Pines, Lori, Pushpa Raja, Nabeel Qureshi, Haiden A. Huskamp, Alisa B. Busch, and Ateev Mehrotra. 2020. "Use of Tele-Mental Health in Conjunction with In-Person Care: A Qualitative Exploration of Implementation Models." *Psychiatric Services* 71 (5): 419–26. https://doi.org/10.1176/appi.ps.201900386.

I'm No Hero

SUZANNE LILKER

In this crazy COVID game
We were never really trained
But quick to be blamed and shamed
I'm no hero

Approached the duty day by day
Through the window on display
People judge and I have no say
I'm no hero

Humbled humiliated can't you see
Behind the masks and PPE
Still alive to collect a fee
I'm no hero

The stakes are high so it makes sense
Emotions sensed to be intense
Egos shattered and in defence
I'm no hero

Infrastructure crumbling
Doors jammed or shutting
Equipment shortages and rationing
Humiliated just for asking
I'm no hero

Taken off of COVID call
Hours and hours not called at all
Code blue or called go intubate
Repeated code whites kept me awake
I'm no hero

Tried to fight it cannot hide it
Lack of control and anxiety
Challenging situations met it seemed
Reliant on a backstabbing team
I'm no hero

Some people think they are the best
But they're no better than the rest
No room to grow or introspect
Growth needs kindness and respect
I'm no hero

No longer considered on front lines
Having flashbacks of those times
Will wish them well
Though they made life hell
I'm no hero

What's more toxic
The virus or the culture?

What gets me back inside those stifling walls
Hello from friendly co-workers in the halls
A grateful patient relieved of pain
The fact that I believe I'm still sane
I'm no hero

We were really put to the test
The truth is we did our best
The usual job is still there with a twist
So do the work and relax the fist
I'm no hero

Note: The line "I'm no hero" is meant to be sung to tune of the line "I'm no Superman" from the theme of the TV show *Scrubs*.

Sidelined by Helen Tang.

Behind the Front Line

(Or, the COVID Experience That Never Was)

RORY O'SULLIVAN

> @snazzyicudoc—24/2/20: Two patients this week with weird diffuse pulmonary embolism #COVID. Same from a buddy in #Kirkland. Anyone else seeing this? This is one funky virus #clot #pandemic

Before the world went sideways, he worried that mediocrity was sneaking up on him.

When he started his career, almost ten years ago, he started with a burst of adrenaline. He was young, sharp, keen, and well trained. He was juggling his way through busy emergency room shifts. He was bouncing around in the back of ambulances in the middle of the night. He was flying into far-flung northern communities, wrapped tightly in Gore-Tex. He was the quintessential swashbuckling TV doctor he had always hoped to be.

Over time, he had grown tired of the night shifts. He had grown weary of the split-second rough-and-tumble of emergency work. He had grown philosophical about the maturity of his craft, about the unglamorous but elemental nature of family medicine. He had moved into urban office practice with purpose and vigor. But here, too, he began to tire. He started to fall out of love with medicine. When he and his wife had a bouncing baby girl, and the opportunity arose to take an extended paternity leave, he leapt at it.

Before the world went sideways, work was the farthest thing from his mind. With months of leave to go, he spent his days changing diapers and pureeing fruit, walking in the park and rhyming off the alphabet.

> @esperanza—4/3/20: So proud to be graduating medical school next month and joining the #front_line in Brooklyn! Dream come true #medstrong #nystrong

> @jonathankaymd—12/3/20: Just finished a week of ICU service #COVID19 #SoCal. Here are my observations re: optimal vent settings and convalescent plasma 1/7

In March, what had started as a social media grumble became a blaring klaxon. When Italy collapsed, and the first cases appeared in Washington State, panic set in fast. The enemy was at the gates. There were the first references to the Great Depression and the Second World War. There were even murmurs of the Black Death. The prime minister was on television, speaking breathlessly. The premier was next, sweating and looking stricken. The first pictures began to filter out of New York. Refrigerator trucks for the bodies. And yet to walk out his front door in Toronto was to step into eerie normalcy. He briefly entertained the thought that the media had worked everyone into a lather, that things were not so bad. Like the rest of the world, he felt numb, knocked about like a buoy in a storm. His whole life, his whole future, lurched to a stop. Wave after wave of cold realizations. One thought rose, again and again, above all the others, unbidden.

He had to go back to work.

How could he not? The stories were coming faster and faster now, of doctors in Wuhan and Spain and their amazing feats of heroism. Working days and weeks on end, isolating from their families, making agonizing ethical choices, some of them struck down in the line of duty. He was not envious, exactly. Perhaps there was a small element of that. It was more that he was wary of his own motivations. He was fearful of being selfish, and lazy. Wasn't medicine a calling, after all? Here was the greatest public health emergency to face the world in generations. How could he look back and explain that he did nothing, he stood quietly by? How could he live with himself?

> @DrAmyLinOhio—21/4/20: to the dude who moved away when I coughed on the bus: Don't worry, I'll still intubate your racist ass when you come to my ER #AsianMed #COVID

> @Frontenac_doc1—18/3/20: volumes are down, never seen the hospital this empty. Is anyone else finding this? Calm before the storm? #COVID19

His day became a hamster wheel of press conferences. As the baby puttered around at his feet, he absorbed the continuous rhythm of updates. The prime minister at 11:30, then the National Task Force at 12:00. The premier at 1:00, and the officer of health at 3:00. The mayor at 3:45. And sometimes, for a bit of colour, the Americans at 5:00. He watched the numbers tick steadily upward, tried to parse the graphs. Began to plan.

Of course, it would be disruptive to go back. His wife was a doctor, already tirelessly adjusting to a new routine of changing clothes at the front door and showering after work. They had elderly parents. They had a responsibility, still fresh, to keep the baby safe. They talked about him living in a hotel. He would have to pick out shoes he could keep at the hospital. He would have to leave all the little touchstones at home: his watch, his wedding ring. He would need freezer bags for his cards and his phone. He got his textbooks out, and his old lecture notes. He imagined himself a boxer in a movie training montage. Mentally running stairs in the chilly pre-dawn air, while theme music swelled around him. What else could he do except be ready?

@frontline_babe—3/4/20: Eight intubations, two codes this shift. Then I drive home and the patio at Applebee's is full! Seething right now. What don't you people understand! #CoronaVirus #stay_home

@graphic_MD—14/4/20: Let's step back and think about why the logarithmic scale is employed in graphs from today's briefing. The logarithmic scale has an interesting history 1/9

In April, the first administrative calls and emails came. The keyword was "redeployment." They were well into lockdown now, and the health-care system like everything else had ground unceremoniously to a halt. There was incredulity as the hospital machine strained at its hinges to keep churning forward, but whispers of "Italy" and "New York" kept much of the complaining at bay. He put his hand up early. He fired off emails, swallowing hard before every final click. I'm ready to come back. I have the training. I have the experience. I'll make the sacrifices. Put me in, Coach.

Finally, he was assigned to a hospital COVID unit as a backup. A second stringer, to be subbed in if the star player twisted his knee. He feasted on the daily emails he was now provided, with the inside track on all the latest medical detail. He drilled, in his head, how to don and doff his protective mask and gown.

@fancy_MDrebel—16/4/20: you guys check out this video—you can turn a shower curtain into a face shield #PPE

@resident_runner—18/4/20: just coded a patient younger than me. Didn't make it. Crappy way to start a shift #COVID19 #medstrong #NHS

Almost immediately, he was besieged by doubt. How long since he had practised such acute medicine? It's one thing to volunteer in truly desperate times, when the ophthalmologists and dermatologists are running the ICU, but was he really qualified now? Was it fair to his family? Was he not committed to caring for his child?

And, sometimes, late at night, he thought about dying. There were more and more memorial tributes spilling out of his social media feeds. Nurses, doctors, old and young. It was not beyond the realm of possibility. What did it say about him, about medicine, that he was usually much more worried about looking silly or unworthy than about the actual physical danger? Still, he began to gently rehearse the letter he would write to his beloved wife and daughter. To be opened in the event of...

@MD_economy—22/4/20: @fordnation #QueensPark needs to pay attention. #COVID19 is a wakeup call that we have failed our most vulnerable #LTC #underhoused #Indigenous.

@Paul_DavidMDMSc—24/4/20 retweeted: watch this infectious disease specialist response to Dr. Oz @ FoxNews. More insane comments!

Even as he imagined himself a casualty of war, the media talk of heroism on the "front line" rankled. It was not that he did not want to think of himself, of doctors, as heroes. Of course this was appealing, and something to which he aspired. But from the inside, he knew it was not that simple. There were a lot of moving parts. There were debates about pay, about equipment, about schedules. There was the discomfort of praise and adulation for sacrifices promised but not yet made.

Morning and night he checked the numbers, trying to predict whether he would be pressed into action. Refresh, refresh, refresh. He watched the cases slowly tick up, and paced the floor. He sat up at night reading emails from professional societies: "Malpractice coverage in the pandemic age," "How to ensure your will is up to date." He cursed whoever decided to send these emails in the evening just before bed. He cursed himself for getting too comfortable, too complacent. He lay awake, and waited.

> @bob_aldernyforsenate—12/5/20: Listen I'm no doctor, but all you medical folks crying on twitter, isn't this what you signed up for? Isn't this why you get paid hundreds of thousands of dollars? #draftdoctors #open_up

> @DrSusanE—12/5/20: @CMA @OMA we need to reimagine medicine from the inside out #COVID19. Time for a paradigm shift that prioritizes #equity #selfcare #socialjustice.

In May, the fog began to lift. The idea that the call to duty might not come began to gain purchase in his head. He was all at once elated and flummoxed. He was not needed. In the greatest medical calamity of his lifetime, the hospital was ticking along just fine without him.

> @liz_bailey—17/5/20: thanks for your kind wishes my daughter is in ICU now we are facing a long night Thank god for FaceTime #thankful Please send your prayers

> @Cowboy_Surgeon—22/5/20: All you snowflakes who can't get through a haircut with your mask on, come talk to me after you've done a 12-hour case in full N95 and face shield #COVID19 #wearamask

Slowly, the world seemed to shake off its cinematic, post-apocalyptic daze and face up to new realities. He was facing up to new realities too. Like everyone anxious to find a *reason*, he cast about for the catharsis, the epiphany, which must come at the end of the tumult. He was learning to let go of the self he had imagined in childhood, the leading man of action, in favour of a new type of role: a supporting character, a family man, with a modern type of masculine sensibility. He began to prepare for a return to the office. He began to think and speak about the next challenges. Depression, anxiety, isolation. Unemployment, poverty, homelessness. Medication shortages, food insecurity. And then, perhaps, the next wave of virus. The work would not be sexy, or fast paced. He would not be eulogized on Twitter, or venerated on Instagram. But there was plenty to do. Sleeves would have to be rolled up.

He no longer worried about the spectre of mediocrity. There were too many other spectres.

@TheRealTrump—25/5/20: We are doing Testing like the world has never seen! Great "reviews"! Many doctors are saying time to get back to NORMAL! Time to do GREAT THINGS! @FoxNews

@DrAmazing—28/5/20: Tough few months. Nice to have staff back in the clinic again. Virtual care is here to stay! Thanks to all for the donations of #PPE ! #MadeinCanada. Bring on #Wave2 Medicine is a calling! #bring_it_on

@SaskMom—22/5/20: Asked my 6 y.o. to draw a picture of superheroes. She drew doctors and nurses in #PPE #thankyouheroes

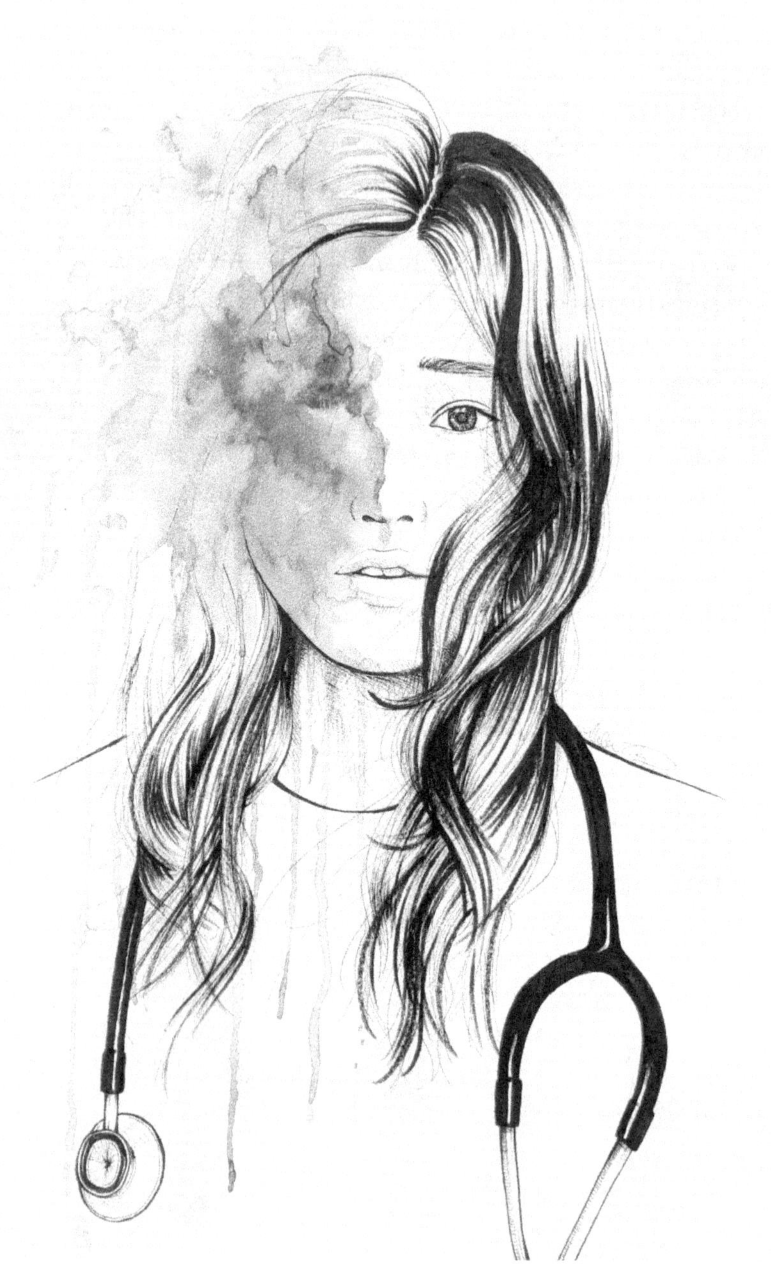

Singularity by Helen Tang.

With Beauty

KACPER NIBURSKI

She smelled different. Something like a promising mango, one that is loose, ripening underneath the fingernails, one that spits black seeds in every bite. Other parts like horse manure.

It started from her head with her hair, tumbled down to her recently shaven legs, anchored itself in her glossy toes that tapped against the Persian, purple carpet we purchased four years ago because of course it would look nice—the place was so empty.

From here, the carpet looked like a bruise. She told me that the hospital was changing slowly, but medical students like myself could still play a role in COVID-19.

"Everyone has their part in making the world whole again," she said.

Her feet stopped fiddling.

"In a pandemic, all the bodies are useful for all the bodies could be no more."

She looked at me, head down, waiting for me to nod.

"This is serious," she said.

I nodded seriously.

Yes, she was right in that there was still magnificence that no one or any thing could take away, that found itself in the flowers from her dress. Yes, she was right that all bodies had use, even as I sat slumped waiting for something more like purpose. Yes, she was right that the world was not whole anymore.

"Yes. I love you and we'll get through this thing," she said.

Her bracelets rattled as she moved her arm around me. She smiled in the soft, infectious way she learned I liked.

Did I smile back? I was not sure. Maybe I winced from the smell.

• • •

I expected a call to arms, a virtual conscription where home was safe while safety was relative. The rules of engagement in this new world were simple: go out to doom oneself to a stranger's careless kindness. Each person was a disease; each encounter was a deadly battle of unknowns. A cough was a snotty punch. A sneeze a spitfire. And a fever prophesied of the heavenly heat to come.

Then it came, a bit lazily, a mere suggestion by the Faculty of Medicine to volunteer with public health agencies. I was to inform that status of patients who had just contracted the virus, dialing into their homes to say that their results were positive. I apologized. I waited. My feet were often draped across my couch during these pauses, blanketed and warm. Her smell nestled itself into the cushions, woken only in my most sporadic movements. Tea was not far away. I sipped it in between the information, the inevitable, and the incredible, until there was total silence.

Hollow whispers followed in each conversation, as though the patient was speaking to their past self and to the person they were now. Then, questions.

How long did the disease last? "From what we understand," I started. How did I get it? "From what you've told me," I continued. What will happen to me? "From what I know," I muddled. "We don't know."

They'd ask who would know. I nearly said her name each time. She was out in the front lines, there among the whirling ventilators that shook against the walls and the bodies that were made to be, as she said, useful. She, who rarefied the invisible. She, who promised to make a cure a balance of optimism and hard work. She was tough. She was strong. She was doing all that could be done for she was to do it all.

I never answered that question; instead, I said we'd call again in a few days. The nights would struggle by, and she would come home almost untouched by the deadened day. She would take a long shower. She would dry off neatly. And after eating a meal I prepared and eyeing me tussle with the dishes, she would tell me that I could not touch her.

"It is a precaution."

Her smell was afresh, different now, like a banana split and beached whale blended together.

"It is a new perfume," she said one day as we ate another meal in silence. "The Chinese apparently tested it against COVID." Some of it still pooled on her neck. The puddle pulsed, pounded.

A text message appeared just before she bit into the lima beans.

"Urgent patient," she said.

I watched her shadow climb the stairs, face lit by the flickers from her phone that could burn everything down, the smell lurking behind like a hungry, bloodied beast.

• • •

She stayed at the hospital longer each day. I took on more shifts of contact tracing. Her delicate laughter slipped into our home late at night when I was already asleep, spent and alone.

When not calling COVID patients, I'd keep the home safe. I cleaned and cleaned and cleaned the surfaces, even if it had no effect on the persistent smell. The carpet was the most difficult, a vortex of cat hair, miscellaneous stains, and uncomfortable furniture-faded purple. Vacuums were no more than loud, chatty animals against its fur. The carpet was too large, too fragile, and too wild to be thrown into a washing machine. Hands would have to work with knees, knees with feet, feet with the earth to scrub and steep and squash and stamp and still, the smell of her lingered. The virus may have been scoured in the Febreze and soap, but the scent transmuted into that rare mix of the first spring blossom and defrosted winter poop.

She failed to notice. She did not remark on the orderliness of the house despite the chaos outside nor of the floor flossed clean nor of the sterility of the place nor of the WASH THE HANDS sign above the kitchen counter nor of how I swore to the virus that I would be its homey arch nemesis nor how I had worn my skin raw by washing my hands so much nor how the welts hurt when I did her dishes nor to the fact that I was helping with her, for her, because of her, cleaning and feeding and calling the countless patients before they would met her healing.

Instead, I caught her in glimpses. She rose before dawn, revealing that there were still things that can break before the horizon. She dressed in more elegant dresses as COVID progressed, despite saying she needed to change into hospital scrubs. Her makeup was perfected into a blend of effortlessness and wide-eyed attention. Her hair curled with delight. She smelt of every wondrous thing crushed, jumbled together.

This is how I would lose her, I told myself. With beauty.

• • •

It was the forty-third time I washed my hands that day. Some of the soap seeped into torn skin. It no longer hurt. A cure was possible, certainly.

I called another patient. They told me that this could not be happening. That this was worse than death. This unknowing.

The door opened. Her form was backlit, unprotected by the night. Another silhouette sniffled near her. Their hips almost touched. He smelled like her.

"This is Cyril. We work together in the ICU."

I nodded seriously.

"I wanted to show him the work you're doing. It's really helping." She smiled as she looked at me.

I nodded seriously.

"Nice to meet you," he said quickly. He went to shake my hand.

I nodded seriously. He outreached further.

"With COVID being so serious, I cannot shake your hand. It is a precaution."

He, too, nodded. She stood at the door. He stood at the door. Their hips got closer, bones and flesh nearly kissing. I could hear the patient on the phone saying, "Hello, Hello, Hello."

I inhaled. What? I inhaled more forcefully, trying to breath in all the air of the home. Nothing.

For the first time during this pandemic, I could not smell a thing.

Management Was Mad

SARAH FRASER

Management was mad
Because there were too many visitors

The patient had a big family
Plus, he was dying

It was COVID times
Yet COVID had not yet come to the community
Maybe the interventions were working

The hospital had a no-child policy
But I saw a girl on the ward one day
She must have sneaked past the red tape
Perhaps a special exemption
It took me by surprise
This tiny human
In such a big, sterile space

His death was coming closer
And management was getting *really* mad
Because family members were sneaking in
Distracting workers at the sign-in desk downstairs
Lying about their identity
So they would have a chance to say goodbye
To their father, brother, friend

I stayed at the hospital late one night
Because I knew his death was coming closer
And I'd have to come back in to the hospital anyway
(for the paperwork, later)

He took his time dying
And I waited for him to do so

Gowned and gloved and masked,
I walked into the room to check on my patient
Still alive.

Ten visitors.
All uncovered people, faces, hands and skin
A nurse popped his head in the room
And told me management was coming
I closed the blinds and door before
stepping out to meet them

"How many people are in there?"
(Management: mad).

We're under the limit, I lied.
"Good."
Good.

Preoccupations of a Public Health Resident

MARISA WEBSTER

The truth is, in this pandemic, I find delight in a bite from a dog with no name. Call it self-pity. Don't get me wrong: I don't wish for Jane, the four-year-old princess, pedalling furiously down 4th Street, hair damp from her morning bath, to start rabidly foaming at the mouth. But it is during these consults that COVID momentarily disappears. Like a book, I can shelve it for later.

"Was the bite provoked?" I ask Jane's father, phone pressed against my cheek.

"Are you implying that it was her fault?" he says sharply. "You think it's her fault."

I imagine a short man on the other end of the line, divorced, with thinning hair—bitter for all these losses.

"That's not what I'm saying."

COVID necessitates that I work from home, alone, slumped over a laptop—a slow, primitive machine on loan from the office. In the time it takes to boot up, I feed the cat, brush my teeth, and watch the night drain away. This is the everyday.

I adjust my light therapy glasses, worn because I am prone to depression, the crushing belief that life will never get better, when sure enough, this second wave only seems to get worse, and I say: maybe there is no end to this? That's how it makes me think at least.

"Look, do you even have kids?" he asks.

Our conversation about rabies has taken a roundabout to reproduction. What I really *want* to say is: you know, buddy, it's none of your business. Instead, as your skillful public health doc, what I really *should* say is: Let's just focus on Jane. She's our priority here. But I don't say either.

"It's complicated," I confess. "Maybe I should just call you back. Is there a good time—"

He blurts out: "My wife died. COVID."

I try to think of something deep or meaningful to offer him—I am a doctor after all—but all that I can muster up is a wimpy "Ohhhh," my voice trailing off, a plume of smoke.

Every morning, I switch my phone number to "Private" so that the people I call can't call me back and mix up their lives with mine. It might sound like strange medicine, but in my world of healing, decisions touch those I will often never see or meet. Yet this seemingly carbon-copy Tuesday has launched me into a life that is sadder than my own.

"I just don't get it. She was young. Thirty-five. Thirty-five! There was nothing wrong with her—she was, she was... everything."

Last night, my husband and I were bickering over greasy fingerprints on the toaster. It's peanut butter, I said. Can't you be more careful? He shrugged, maybe even rolled his eyes. The mob in me started to protest. Standing there I thought, I could kill him. Not really, but you know how these battles go; a five-dollar condiment becomes larger than life. But now my reasoning seems shaky; my logic a little muddy. The fingerprints on the toaster—at the time a small torment—now feel like a small blessing.

I watch the marmalade-coloured leaves float past the window. I can almost smell their musky sweetness, the sign of another imminent ending. Jane's father is quiet on the line. I don't know what to say or even how to go about saying it. Unlike the public health journals that I read, there is no methods section in life. We make things up as we go along: we hope that our tomatoes won't rot; that our luggage arrives on time. We do the best with what we have.

Today I sit in silence with a stranger. I don't ask him to be anywhere other than where he is in his grief and his sorrow. And in some sense, he does the same for me. This is service; a connection between equals. It is the only way to navigate this uncharted territory—this pandemic—for which there seems to be no clear path.

Bongo Guy in Lockdown

CHRISTOPHER BLAKE

I like bongo music as much as the next guy.

Its warm tones are the soundtrack to a thousand sunny summer days, the score to countless campfire nights. It calls to mind friends and family, a carefree time and place where the drinks are flowing and the smell of food fills the air. You would think, then, that the bongo would be the perfect antidote to the woes of lockdown life, harkening back to a happier, healthier time.

You would think that and you would be wrong. So very, calamitously, wrong.

But I get ahead of myself. Allow me, if you will, to set the stage for the drama yet to unfold.

In 2018 I moved in to the top two floors of a triplex in a leafy Toronto neighbourhood. The apartment was a private paradise with turn-of-the-century charm and all the modern amenities a discerning millennial could hope for. Big bay windows let in light filtered through stately trees and functional air conditioning broke the heat of sweltering summers. In short, it offered everything I had vainly sought from the ten apartments I had lived in over the ten preceding years. Finally, here was a house that I could call home.

And at first the neighbourhood truly was as perfect as it had seemed. In the mornings I went for runs along the lakeshore. In the evenings I strolled the bustling main street with its hipster restaurants and little free libraries. In those heady early days, I'd repeat inanely to my partner that it was as if some sentient AI had scanned my brain and manifested a community tailor-made for my quirks and eccentricities. I mean, three used bookstores and an indie movie theatre? Come on! I now know that these early gambits were merely a trap, that, without realizing, I was being lured deeper and deeper into a labyrinth from which madness was the only escape.

For the first year, that glorious bygone age when I was lulled into a false sense of security, the house next door sat empty. I was told that the owner planned to renovate and then re-list at a higher price but no construction ever happened. Through dusty windows I looked in on empty rooms lit by strange red lights, as if the homeowners were staging some obscure art show I was too provincial to appreciate. The street was quiet, practically bucolic. The idyllic silence was interrupted only by the joyful laughter of children or the pleasant ringing of a bicycle bell.

And then, one day, a moving van pulled up next door. I couldn't have known it then, but this inauspicious development heralded the arrival of the greatest threat my sanity had yet to face. Had I known then what I know now, would I have stayed?

No, I would not have.

Had I known then what I know now, I would have shorted the stock market and stocked a cabin deep in the Ontario wilderness with three years' worth of supplies and bongo resistant sound-proofing. But time makes fools of us all and hindsight is, as they say, twenty-twenty.

It started innocently enough. On sunny days, the rhythm of the bongo would blow through our open windows with the breeze, seeming to capture and distill the careless summer sun. Back then, the drumbeat came mostly in the weekend daytime, a perfectly respectable time for bongo music. Did I ever reach a state of pique when the incessant, monotonous drumbeat stretched from minutes to hours then through the whole afternoon?

Yes.

But back then the bongo was not inescapable. I had a whole city to explore: restaurants to visit, art galleries to attend, trails to hike. Back then my world had not yet collapsed to the size of an eleven hundred square foot apartment and a hundred square foot deck repurposed by local raccoons as the communal latrine. It never occurred to me that one day I might be trapped and forced to listen, day in and day out, to the sort of monster that would play the same continuous bongo refrain for five straight hours. Those were more innocent days.

In early March, when the coronavirus hit North America in earnest, my new schedule left me working in the hospital every two weeks out of three and from home the third week. At first, I savoured the thought of working from home. I would listen to '70s Japanese jazz piano and sip smoky teas from my Hawaiian volcano mugs while wearing slippers I'd pilfered from the Fairmont Banff Springs. I had even laid away a respectable, though not obscene, store of toilet paper. Could one ask, global pandemic notwithstanding, for anything more?

But, alas, it was not to be, for I was not the only one harried by fate to work from home. Inspired, perhaps, by these dark hours of humanity, unshackled by an abundance of free time, and fortified, no doubt, by the sort of high-grade hallucinogens necessary to power a six-hour bongo solo, the Bongo Guy was born.

My partner and I call him the Bongo Guy though we do not know their gender. Amidst the fog of war, one must imagine one's enemy to better comprehend them, so that one day, perhaps, they may be overcome. But, amidst the terrible depths of the pandemic, when all seemed lost and there was no past and no future (only one burning, continuous, now) I did not believe that the Bongo Guy *could* be overcome.

His persistence was relentless. His disregard for the well-being of his community was boundless. His ability to play the same dum-dum/dum-dum over and over again was unmatched by any force short of a metronome. What was I to a power such as this? How could I contend with the sheer anarchic madness of a man who wanted nothing more than to watch the world burn, one bongo note at a time?

His grim, funereal dirge dragged on through cold and through heat, through snow and through rain. Faced with the incomprehensible, the human mind struggles to rationalize events with the basic rules of the universe. If only I could understand Bongo Guy, perhaps I could withstand him too.

Perhaps Bongo Guy was newly unemployed and bored witless, the bongo his only outlet. Perhaps, amidst the chaos of the world, the repetitive drone of the bongo allowed Bongo Guy to approach a state of semi-nirvana, like a Tibetan monk at prayer. Perhaps Bongo Guy was simply smoking copious amounts of weed. To this day, I cannot say.

My partner, working from home every day rather than every third week, bore the brunt of his relentless assault. Though in the hospital I gowned and gloved, masked and face-shielded, for her there was no personal protective equipment to defend against the Bongo Guy's onslaught. At night, after I'd flense my skin of hospital germs with scalding water and drying soap, I'd lay face down on the couch, exhausted, and hear, as if on some devilish cue, the Bongo Guy begin to play.

It would go on for hours, past the bedtime of small children, past, indeed, my own bedtime.

dum-dum
dum-*dum*
dum-DUM
DUM!-DUM!

My partner and I would lay awake in bed, cursing him, trying to imagine how a person could go on playing like this, how a neighbourhood could go on listening to it. And then, just when things seemed at their darkest, an unlikely hero arose.

It was late, nearly 10 o'clock (on a school night) and dusk had settled upon our shaded street. And still, the Bongo Guy droned on. It had been this way for hours, hours which felt like geological ages of the earth. All I wanted was the sweet release of sleep. Was that too much to ask? Was I being punished for something I had done in some horrible past life? Was all of this (the pandemic, the bongos), some sort of demented Twilight Zone reject episode I'd somehow stumbled into?

And then it happened.

The Bongo Guy droned on, wild, insatiable, and then a voice rang out from across the street, rang out in the clear, indignant tones of a man, trying his best to be civil, pushed past any human's breaking point.

"BONGO GUY! SHUT. UP."

The bongo stopped. My partner and I looked at one another as silence fell like snowfall over the street. Was this the end? Had it been this easy all along? Was a single chastening really enough to end our lockdown nightmare?

I was elated, not merely by the end of the musical torture but by the shared humanity I'd felt when I'd heard the other man call out the rogue musician. He too, had named him Bongo Guy, though presumably he knew no more of his gender or his life than we did. He too had listened for months to the relentless bongo drone, likely complaining to his own partner, until, finally, he too had snapped. In that moment, amidst the grim isolation of the pandemic, I felt, finally, a sense of human communion. I felt, perhaps, that humanity might make it through this global catastrophe after all.

Bongo Guy was silent for the rest of that week. The next time I heard him play, perhaps a week later, he lacked the verve and stamina that had been his hallmark. He played for perhaps thirty listless minutes but I could tell his heart wasn't in it.

A few weeks after that, perhaps trying out a different tack, he broke out in a new and more experimental tune, finally diverging from his monotonous dum-dum/dum-dum into something resembling music. This, too, was short lived. Perhaps sensing a vacuum to be filled, some neighbourhood miscreant began practicing their recorder with riotous abandon but I think even they understood how pale a replacement they made and I never heard them play again.

Time passes. Summer has come. The thermometers have cracked thirty degrees nearly every day. It is, to coin a phrase, bongo weather. How pleasant it would be to open a window and hear again the easy thrum of bongo music on the air. And yet, Bongo Guy is silent. The world has opened up again and Bongo Guy too has moved on, perhaps playing his bongos now at an overcrowded beach or in Trinity Bellwoods Park.

I did not shout him down and yet I feel I bear some blame for his silence. We were all thinking it. It just happened that another, braver man than I scarified himself for all of us. In that sacrifice, I found again the sense of community that was lost when we were forced indoors by a virus. In that sacrifice, I learned that we were not alone.

For that reason, if for no other, Bongo Guy will always have my thanks. He reminded us, in our darkest hour, that no man is an island, that we are, all of us, one big, dysfunctional, family. And, when I move this summer into the countryside, an acre of land between me and the nearest house, I will look back on those pandemic days when I was driven nearly mad by the Bongo Guy as a time when all of us were alone and all of us were together.

Mango Season

ARUNDHATI DHARA

Every year, just before my birthday, the Alphonso mangoes are in season. Known scientifically as *Mangifera indica*, its real name is the King of Mangoes. This is not hyperbole, as Alphonsos are truly the ruler of all fruit. When people who have travelled to India wax poetic about the colours and tastes being somehow more intense, in that smug self-congratulatory way they do, make no mistake they are referring to the Alphonso mango.

The fruit is small, fitting easily in the palm of my hand. The skin is nondescript but inside is a gaudy, embarrassing orange. Smooth, silky flesh gives way to a slender seed. The juice drips from your fingers and the pieces slip in your hands. If you eat this mango, you will be ruined. You will crave the taste all year, waiting until you might have it again. Do not confuse The King with the imposter Ataulpho variety. That is fool's gold. I have heard in whispers there are mangoes from Pakistan that rival the Alphonso. I am not convinced this is possible, and in any event, I am a faithful woman. As evidence of the Alphonso's superiority, I understand there is a black market for them in Detroit. They are smuggled in from Windsor because they are prohibited in the United States, lest they infect domestic mangoes with whatever fruit ailments they might carry. I think the Americans are just afraid of a far superior product.

I spent Alphonso season in the hospital. We wore scrubs and masks to see patients. Each day, I arrived in workout gear and large-framed glasses, adding scrubs in that particular drab green meant to reduce eye strain. I slid a black bandana over my black hair and a blue mask over my nose and mouth and went upstairs to see patients. I looked like any of the swarms of doctors and nurses, identical at first glance except for the dark skin of my hands and forehead. I was embarrassed that I could not identify one nurse from another—nurses I have worked with for almost a decade.

The diagnoses on my daily patient lists varied. One was admitted for heart failure because they didn't get immediate care for the heart attack they probably had in the early days of COVID. Another had been quietly declining at home and was just no longer able to cope on their own. Their children and spouses and dogs and cats would be waiting when I entered, on phones and tablets and phablets, expecting. They were nothing but talking heads on screens that weren't quite big enough to catch their ears and the tops of their heads. I was nothing but a forehead and eyes behind a mask and a face shield. Sometimes we talked about how well their mothers or husbands were doing and when they might go home. There was always some panic. The hospital was not safe: it was full of COVID (it wasn't, objectively, but that didn't actually matter). But home was also not safe. It was full of...nothing. Just solitude. The aloneness was a horror.

The irony was that by Alphonso season there were no COVID patients admitted to our hospital. My patients were the collateral damage of the COVID pandemic, not counted in the daily statistics, but somehow just as tragic. Still, COVID was the only thing anyone talked about. How many cases today? Where were they? How many deaths nationally? Are you going on vacation? Do you know if school will open again this year? What if we have a superspreader? Did you hear about what happened in NYC? Information was king—even if it was only rumour or conjecture.

We moved to Canada when I was only a baby, and my parents set about trying to recreate the flavours they knew in a foreign country. They were committed cooks, but the flavours prized in Canadian produce were decidedly underappreciated in our household. Spicy, sour chutneys ruled our kitchen. Unable to find what she wanted at the supermarket, my mother ventured outside our apartment, in full view of all six lanes of the Don Valley Parkway South, and picked crabapples to make chutney, because it was the sourest thing she could lay hands on in Toronto. My parents rode buses and trains to source the vegetables they craved from small, poky shops we have called "The Indian Store" ever since. The vegetables from the regular supermarket were quite literally referred to as "chappa" or "tasteless." So when my father, years after arriving in Toronto, found an Alphonso mango, he had no choice but to buy it. The price was obscene but he had discovered gold. The mangoes were sometimes underripe when he brought them home, but it didn't matter. We would carefully place them in the buckets with our rice for a few days, removing them when the entire kitchen was filled with a distinctive sweet smell.

Since I moved away from home, my father has made it his business to supply me with Alphonso mangoes. He has travelled on airplanes with suitcases filled with one pair of pants and three boxes of mangoes. Once a security officer opened the suitcase, looked at the boxes of mangoes, filling Pearson with their smell, and closed it again, nodding in understanding. He has driven for hours to deliver them to me—in pelting rain—a postal service for fruit. Every year, he tells me how much my grandfather loved mangoes, how and when he ate them, how he and his siblings picked them from trees as children, how they were cut and served to the family, and about the particular varieties that grew where he lived.

My children love mangoes. When my father's boxes arrive, they can disappear in a matter of hours if I don't hide them.

With the narcissism of childhood, they know these mangoes are just for them. I know I should be happy to give my children whatever gives them joy but what I really want to do is tell them they all rotted and then eat them all in secret. This plan would be perfect, except that they can smell the ripening mangoes in the rice buckets. I hold back the beasts by telling them the mangoes aren't quite perfect yet.

At night, when they are sleeping, I lift the lid and investigate. If a fruit smells particularly good I cut it open and eat it. (I tell myself I need to test them for the children, after all.) There is an art to cutting a mango. Sliding the knife along the seed to maximize the two large pieces gives you a thin mango slice, the centre of which is the seed itself. Two cuts along the sides of this disc and you're left with the seed and four satisfying pieces of fruit.

When I was small it was a great treat to eat the seed, called the tenkai. There was always plenty of mango flesh on it, and as a child you could squish and squeeze every last drop out of it with your hands and mouth and make a giant mess. Standing over my kitchen sink with the seed, I take a bite and close my eyes. Alphonsos taste cartoonish. They are laughably sweet with some vague vanilla flavour. When ripe they have no tartness at all, but if you aren't careful the flesh slides down your throat so fast you never get to taste it. This is a tragedy to be avoided at all costs. Leaning into the counter, dripping mango juice into the sink, I like to think I look more dignified now. I am sure I am wrong.

In the morning, my children ask about the mangoes, and once given the go-ahead they eat them all day until they are gone. Then they ask for more. "But they're all done," I answer. "You ate them." To my great horror, I have discovered that my children have no standards when it comes to mangoes. No Alphonso? No problem. Apparently frozen mangoes suffice.

This year, there were no Alphonsos. COVID stopped the flow of goods into Pearson and my parents couldn't come to see me anyway. We had only endless bags of frozen mangoes. Perhaps as some kind of penance, I ate them almost daily through the pandemic season. They are only mango-approximates, and in May, they tasted like grief.

The worst cases were when patients were dying and brothers and sisters and sons and daughters had to decide who would be designated as a visitor. Even after the early restrictions eased, two visitors were allowed only after a patient had been deemed to be actively dying. This phrase might seem like an oxymoron, but trust me, there are things that happen—sometimes more or less quickly—in a prescribed order. I never asked how families made these decisions because I couldn't imagine a good answer. How would I respond to "I'm here because I was mom's favourite"?

Some families would smuggle in more than two visitors at night, and nursing staff would just find three children curled up with the patient in the morning. My favourite families were the ones who ignored the regulations altogether. They'd have food, and chatter, and hug one another, reminding us of what we are supposed to do when people are dying. Those families were very clear that there wouldn't be a funeral—what would be the point? They'd have a big party when this mess was over and celebrate like Grandma would have wanted them to. They'd offer me cookies, but I couldn't smell them behind my mask and in any event, I no longer ate at the hospital. By the time I had sanitized, removed the mask and the shield, re-sanitized my hands, the surfaces, my food, and maybe offered sanitizer to a passing phlebotomist for good measure, I had no appetite at all.

In August my aunt was admitted to the hospital. The quarantines stopped me from going to Toronto. In any event, it turned out we were a "rules" family; only my cousin went to the hospital. No one had seen my aunt for months due to COVID regulations, and when she was in the hospital, we swarmed like very annoying fruit flies. We buzzed with texts and earless phablet heads. She didn't have COVID. We didn't actually know what happened except that she collapsed. Every test they ran was negative, and within a few days she was back to her stubborn self. We were all relieved. The day she was discharged, my cousin made sure she ate, played her favourite prayer and settled her in bed. She was gone ten minutes later.

I watched the funeral on my computer, my mother weeping, one uncle's voice cracking as he sang a bajan, an aunt speaking with the rushed breathy voice of grief. All the chairs were six feet apart. My family generally followed the protocols, sitting six feet away from one another. My parents moved their chairs close together.

A botanist by training, my father's PHD dissertation was about some kind of cotton disease that devastated farmers in India. I'm not sure whether it's the chicken or the egg, but my father can also grow anything. Over the years he has collected the seeds of vegetables you've never heard of, carefully scraping them out before drying and storing them. Despite his bad knees, he has grown bitter gourds and chili peppers and varieties of cucumbers that make the very best chutney. He has even, by some miracle, grown sour green leaves that are spiced and pickled between the concrete pavers on the patio. They come up every year. I, on the other hand, have killed mint, well known among gardeners to be "unkillable."

My dad said, "She could grow anything." The pear tree in my aunt's backyard was always heavy with fruit. Sometimes she would ride the 53 Steeles East bus to our house with a bag full of perfect pears, oh so slightly underripe (just how I like them). As a child I would pick the pears from her tree, taking one bite and throwing them away if they weren't perfect, trying not to get caught wasting all the fruit like an idiot. My father has never grown any fruit in his garden. I'm not sure if this is because he can't do it or it can't be done. I am a little afraid to ask because I am very likely to get a lesson in the micronutrient requirements of fruit in soil, root depth, and other incomprehensible minutiae. My aunt would have cared about the science of plants, though she was not trained in it. I only wanted to eat pears.

Next year, I will have my first garden. I am trying to convince my father to teach me to grow all the vegetables he does, but he seems reluctant. I think when I killed the mint, I disappointed him. I expect we'll still have COVID so I might not get my Alphonsos for a second year. I am determined not to eat frozen mangoes, however, so I have decided to plant a pear tree. The king is dead. Long live the king.

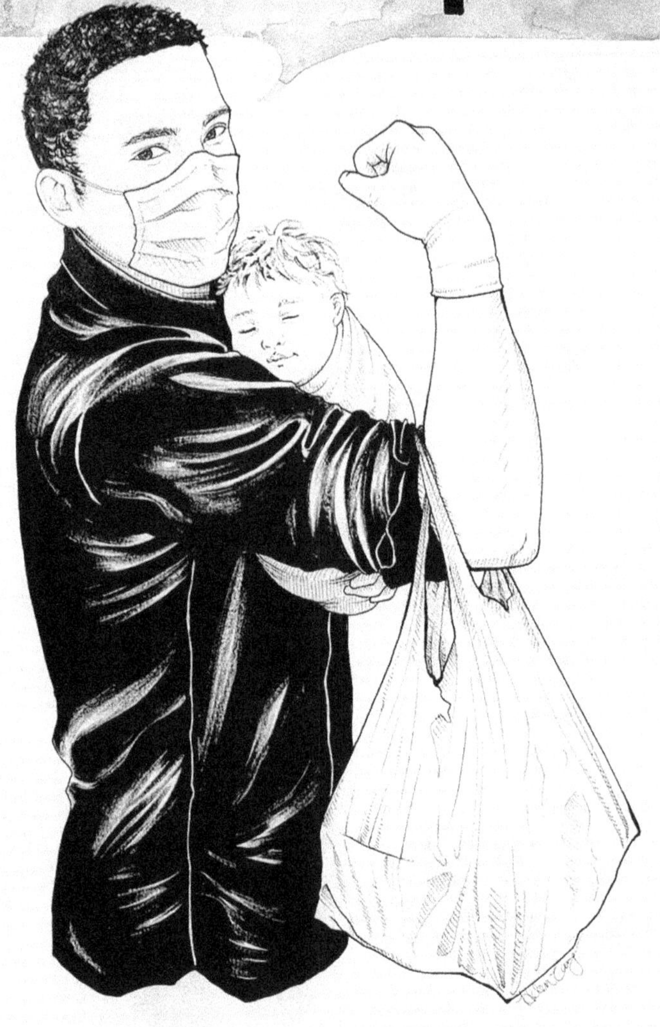

Solidarity by Helen Tang.

I Am Letting Myself Go

(Or, Humans of Late COVID)

ELIZABETH NIEDRA

In the caverns and crevices of my living room, I have nothing
    else to do
I am letting myself go.

My eyebrows like startled gremlins march in little armies
    across the space above my eyes
It will be wild bush, it will be metal scrub brush sludge, it will be
    hedge-mazes of electrocuted porcupines
I will be my father, I will be myself but ugly boy, before their
    march is finalized
I am letting myself go

I coat my fingertips with toxic neon cheddar dust
Mine the bag like a rude raccoon, cover the earth with radioac-
    tive finger marks
I crush lightning bolts between my teeth, just watch me crunch
    crunch crunch
I am letting myself GO

I'll wait until my hair is long, too long to hide or pin or shape
I will slick it back upon my head, like a gangster, like a rat
Like demon woman, outer space
I will lead the revolution
NO—MORE—HARD—PANTS
No more pants of any shape
Only zig-zags and rabbit feet and Dorito crumbs and rage
I with dress myself in balloons 'til I am fat and bubbly like a grape
Hike my sweatpants to my armpits so you believe I have no waist
I AM LETTING GO

Of monkeys on my aching back who pick boldness from my hair
Of hypocrites who walk like gods, and talk like gods, and speak for God but are likely going—well, you know where
No more rules except the ones I'm makin' up, this is Jumanji on a dare
Because why? Because you know why
Look around
And I mean this with love
But who fucking cares.

I am go

To walk on lava, soar off ledges, flying squirrel king
Tap dance with cartoon rabbits out on Saturn's farthest rings

I am go into the vacuum where no space or time exists
I am go, beyond the great beyond, where loneliness, destruction, understanding, fear, fraternity, learning how to sew, unlearning everything and I mean everything, relearning everything and I mean everything, can we put this back together, will anything ever be, again, or is this how it all begins to end, where all that sits.

I am go out to the swamp at midnight
Screaming at my own moon, yeah

I am
Sitting silent, by myself, off my phone, with my thoughts
So quiet, by the kitchen stair
I am
I am, staying there.

Life and Death in Denendeh

EWAN AFFLECK

Underfoot the spring snow is crisp in the morning; it will soften later in the day as the temperature rises. Little rivulets of melt-water course down the steeper sections of the trail, a film of ice made overnight forming a translucent skin over the rushing water. The ice shatters easily to my boot, with a wet almost guilty crunch.

The dogs are muzzle down, feverishly tracking stories left in fresh prints; fox, rabbit, coyote, I guess. They find joy in a tumult of smells that I cannot imagine. They dig in moist soil exposed after a long winter dormant, pausing to sample earth with avid noses, pursuing a narrative that is wholly hidden to me, a social media born of instinct and urine.

Soon the trail widens and simple white wooden crosses can be seen through the trees. In the spring of 2021, I was drawn back to this place, returning almost daily to walk the dogs and enjoy the quiet. This plot of earth served as the burial ground for early residents of the newly founded city of Yellowknife; between 1938 and 1946 almost forty people were buried in the sandy berm. Their names, dates of death, and ages are noted on a sign erected by the city. Almost all were men, and many were very young: 25, 28, 30, 30, 22, 17, 22 years of age. There are also many children; only six of those buried in the cemetery lived past the age of fifty years, only two past sixty. The city of Yellowknife was founded in the 1930s by prospectors seeking the promise of gold. The first gold mine opened on September 5, 1938, twelve days before a twenty-five-year-old miner named Art McIntyre became the first person buried in the cemetery.

The graveyard sits in a ravine between two broken and worn granite bluffs that cradle a forest of black spruce and birch. The rock is textured with black and green lichen that mark the passage of time. Over the months of winter, a little stream deliberately builds a thick shelf of ice across the floor of the ravine with successive layers of overflow. This natural passageway marks a traditional Dene portage between Great Slave Lake and Long Lake to the west. A sign in the cemetery suggests that Elders believe that, long before the city was founded, the area served as a burial ground for local Indigenous people.

I had moved to Yellowknife in 2001, another non-Indigenous physician from the south seeking gratification; twenty years later the North had become home. In the spring of 2021, the COVID-19 virus—which a year before had rapidly reframed global commerce, travel, and assembly—remained a theoretical construct for those of us in the Northwest Territories. There had been scant infections over the preceding year, no major illness, and no death. Public health efforts that were rigorously followed at the outset of the pandemic had become nostalgic customs with feeble adherence; COVID, much like Godot, never seemed to arrive. Residents returned to pubs and coffee shops, and congregated in each other's houses, the threat seemingly vanquished. In the lull, local physicians took to bickering amongst themselves about the true threat of the virus, some arguing that COVID was more damaging as an artifact that infringed on social liberties than as a threat to corporal well-being. Premasticated social media fueled debates over conjecture and spilt beer, as the news of the world filtered into our isolated bubble as through a periscope; Italy, New York City, India, and Brazil assumed dimensions of academic curiosity. Our capacity to believe that misfortune will spare us is transcendent, and when it does not result in death, can spare us a miserable existence.

In 1928, ten years before Art McIntyre was buried in the Yellowknife cemetery, a Hudson's Bay Company supply ship, the SS *Distributor*, made its annual trip down the Mackenzie River. The *Distributor* was a 150-foot steamship acquired by the Hudson's Bay Company to carry cargo from the south to remote trading posts along the Mackenzie River. Fort Providence, Fort Simpson, Fort Good Hope, place names that speak of contemporary history. In recent years, there has been a movement to repatriate traditional place names, Zhahti Koe, Liidlii Kue, Radeyilikoe. Place names tell a worthy story if you listen; the Northwest Territories declares a very different history than Denendeh, the land of the people. The Mackenzie was named for a Scottish explorer who "discovered" a river that was already known as the Dehcho, the Big River.

The Dehcho runs like a great artery through the heart of Denendeh, and in the summer of 1928 the SS *Distributor* carried a terrible payload. Stopping at each trading post to discharge goods for the year, the ship rode the current downstream. Within days of the *Distributor*'s visit, local people began to fall ill with cough, shortness of breath, and fever. The crew of the boat carried a particularly virulent strain of influenza, which they unwittingly spread with their commerce.

Dene with living memory of the time are now mostly gone, but Elders speak of stories passed down to them of entire families and communities falling ill, of scores of dead, of those who did not fall ill digging day and night to bury family and friends; bodies would be wrapped in simple blankets and sometimes placed two to a grave to save time. Many families abandoned their traditional summer fishing camps and escaped into the bush to isolate themselves from illness.

Some suggest this was a recrudescence of the Spanish flu, an exceptionally deadly strain of the H1N1 influenza virus that swept across the globe ten years earlier, killing tens of millions worldwide; but this is conjecture. Travel to Denendeh was still quite limited in 1928, and once introduced the virus found a fertile home among a people with limited immunity and few resources to combat the illness. A virtual absence of medical services at the time helped fuel a high death rate.

In 1928 the non-Indigenous presence in Denendeh was principally in the form of the iconic Canadian colonial triumvirate: clergy, the Royal Canadian Mounted Police, and Hudson's Bay Company staff. Many years would pass before the Canadian government invested in public health services for Indigenous people in Canada's North, and the impetus was not human rights, inclusivity, or altruism but the Cold War.

Indigenous Peoples, living independently in what recent interlopers had chosen to call Canada, unwittingly became pawns in a game of international sovereignty. After the Second World War, a paranoid imperialism on the part of Russia and the United States fueled great interest in the land and ocean that lay between them. The construction of the Distant Early Warning, or DEW, Line, a series of radar stations installed by the Americans across the North American Arctic to intercept Russian nuclear missiles directed at the United States, prompted unprecedented activity in northern Canada. The Canadian government feared losing claim to hitherto superfluous tracts of land in the far north. What better way to assert your sovereignty over the land than to claim the people living there as Canadian citizens? Citizenship was rapidly conferred on Indigenous Peoples in the Arctic, and was accompanied by family allowance, housing and health services, as well as forced resettlement, residential schooling, and starvation.

The first COVID death in the Northwest Territories occurred in August 2021, eighteen months after the declaration of the pandemic, and after about four and a half million people had died worldwide. The delta variant had found its way to a remote community, where people had gathered to play traditional Dene hand games. The virus quickly spread through the hamlet, and followed visitors home to neighbouring communities. A few individuals became quite ill, requiring hospitalization at Stanton Territorial Hospital in Yellowknife, where I work as a physician.

Death is a common narrative in hospitals; by modern medical custom it is compartmentalized and sanitized by protocol, emotional distance, and technology. The curation of care is designed to promote a mythology that Western medicine can somehow evade mortality, a ruse perpetuated by removing death from the community and sequestering it inside institutional walls. The hospital in Yellowknife serves this institutional purpose well; it sits like a fortress, blasted into Precambrian rock, long sterile hallways adorned with hundreds of security cameras that monitor for potential intruders. Automatic doorways open exclusively to security fobs, obstructing access to community members. What is advertised as a place of healing, where family and person and culture and community can congregate to nourish well-being, bristles against trespassers. The North is a friendly and welcoming place, but culture and community are not meant to breach these walls; they are intruders.

The global scope of the pandemic belies the singular act of dying from the virus. While oddly pedestrian, the loss of my first patient to COVID was also unnervingly dreamlike. The end of life is a community event for the Dene. It is not unusual to have crowds of family and community members spilling out into the hospital hallway as an Elder approaches the end of their time. An encampment in a foreign edifice; a resilient expression of tradition enduring in a parched landscape, resolute and determined. Food is shared, stories told, and time is patiently passed. I have never really understood the language of these gatherings, and to this day feel like a foreign agent trespassing on a sacred ceremony when I enter the room on my daily rounds. Stripped of artifice, I stumble in my medical idiom to speak of the patient's condition, as all eyes in the room pause to listen, revealing in their silence how truly disconnected I am from what is really happening.

Death from COVID is a far more solitary journey. No family, no community can attend. Imprisoned by the virus, a patient is captive, breathless, in a private universe, visited only by medical personnel cloaked in protective shrouds that obscure expressions of warmth and compassion. Scattershot sound and video through a cellphone to a desperate family in a remote community seems to accentuate the void. There is a sense of powerlessness one has in caring for an individual dying of COVID. The routine armamentarium of tools available to combat illness are impotent. Time alone becomes the metre of success or failure.

A few days after the death, I returned to the Yellowknife cemetery, accompanied by the dogs. It had been almost three months since our last visit to the ravine. The ground was no longer sodden from the spring melt, but dry, and the earth on the trodden path was cracked and fissured in places.

I set out with some trepidation, as the summer months in Yellowknife are known for plentiful mosquitoes that make misery of hikes in the bush. But the heat of the summer tempers the load, and by August, time in the bush is usually more tolerable. Further, I would bear the inconvenience of mosquitoes for a moment of quiet in the cemetery and the history it spoke and wisdom it held.

After twenty minutes, I reached the bottom of the ravine, where the forest thins out; the white crosses soon came into view. Grass that had grown around them was now yellowing and dry. I had the impression that no one had visited in months.

The sign listing the names and ages of those interred remained in place, unmolested. On the sign is a reproduction of an old photograph taken in March 1946. The image shows a Catholic priest, bearded with open Bible in hand, standing at the head of a casket adorned with flowers. He is facing the camera and appears to be reading, performing the three sacraments of the last rites, I imagine. On either side of the casket stand two young Indigenous men in profile, finely dressed, heads bowed, lips closed, and arms pressed to their bodies, listening. The earth around the casket has been disturbed; there is snow on the hill behind them. The caption under the photograph reads, "Edward and Bud Lessard stand over the casket of brother Raymond at Back Bay Cemetery, 1946."

I tried to imagine the ceremony, a sombre gathering for one so young. In March the wind off the lake would still have been bitter, cooled by fast ice. I imagine the casket had been transported across the bay by dog team. A path then led up to the gravesite, the trodden snow dirtied by the boots of men. The ground would have been hard, unforgiving and very, very cold. I paused and studied the white crosses. The granite bluffs had born witness—recent in the scale of their age—but kept their own council. Silence had long supplanted voices.

We are poor students of history in the digital age, distracted by feral effluent from invasive media that tethers us to set belief. We are so habituated to unbroken stimulation that inaction and quiet become a source of discomfort. History in our age is eroding before a welter of superficial clatter. To be impoverished of history is to be impoverished of wisdom.

Raymond Lessard was seventeen years of age at the time of his death. He was born in 1929, a year after the great influenza pandemic had come to Denendeh, when life was more fragile, infectious disease was largely incurable, and vaccines were in their infancy. A continent and an ocean away, while scores of Dene lay dying of influenza in 1928, the Scottish physician Sir Alexander Fleming first observed penicillin.

We adapt rapidly to that which had formerly seemed miraculous. The suggestion that one could swallow a little capsule filled with inert grains of powder to kill offensive germs invading the body, or activate an internal arsenal of humoral agents to ward off infectious threat by depositing a drop of fluid beneath the skin, would have seemed delusional through most human

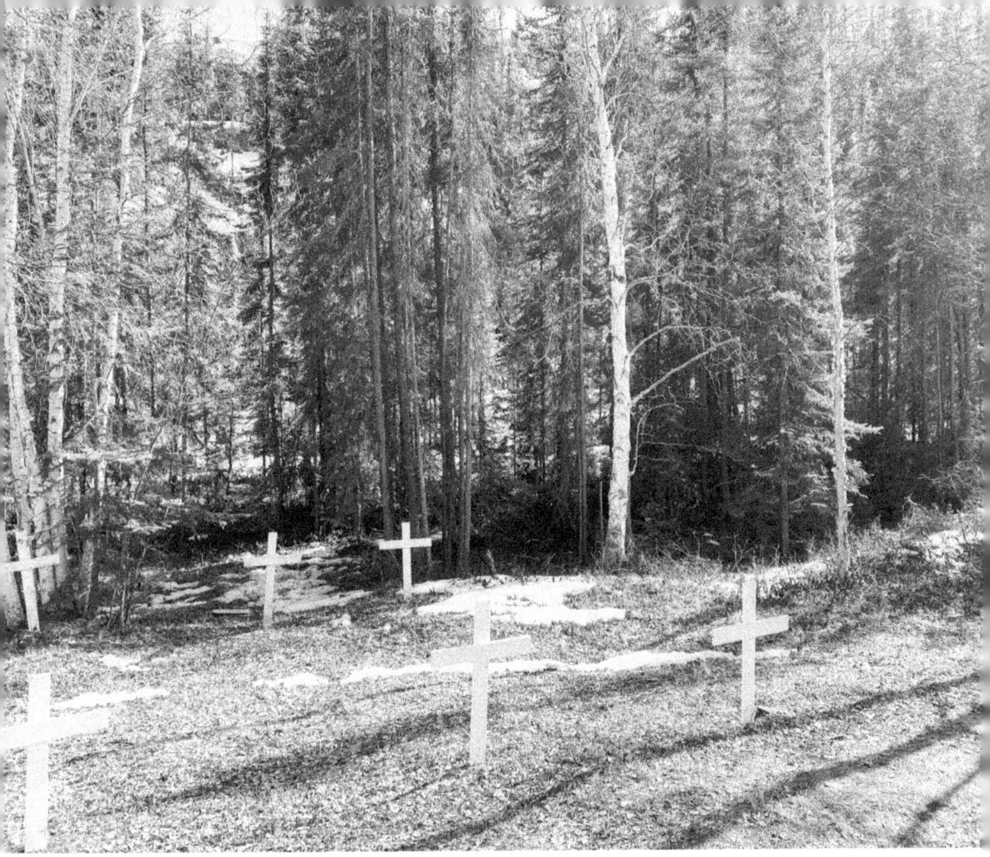

Back Bay Cemetery, Yellowknife. (Photo by Ewan Affleck.)

history. But amazement is soon replaced by entitlement; we are lulled into a sense of mastery over life by the magic of our achievements. COVID has threatened that mastery, revealing fissures in our control and sense of order. But it also normalizes our place on Earth.

Almost a century has passed between the great flu epidemic of 1928 and the arrival of COVID in Denendeh. While we cry for the individual who dies and feel sorrow for those left sundered, there is an unruffled dignity to the cycle. The symmetry of these events—spanning almost a century—was somehow comforting.

A moment passed, in grace, in equanimity. Then I called to the dogs, turned, and we headed back up the path between the birch, black spruce, and soft granite hills.

Jipasi na'sɨk melkitai

TANAS SYLLIBOY

Jipasi, I am afraid to face this virus
Jipasi, I am afraid for our youth
Jipasi, I am afraid for our elders
Jipasi, I am afraid for our language
Jipasi, I am afraid we will be forgotten
Jipasi, I am afraid we will be left behind

Melkitai, I am brave to face this virus
Melkitai, I am brave because of our youth
Melkitai, I am brave because of our elders
Melkitai, I am brave because of our language
Melkitai, I am brave to never be forgotten
Melkitai, I am brave to never be left behind

Mi'kmaw translation:
Jipasi: I am afraid
Melkitai: I am brave
Jipasi na'sɨk melkitai: Afraid but I am brave

In the ER, Patients Need My Comfort But I Am Scared to Give It

SARAH-TAÏSSIR BENCHARIF

As an emergency physician, I talk about life and death often, but never like this.[1]

I met Mrs. B in the emergency department where she was sent with a sore throat and cough. There was a COVID-19 outbreak in her retirement home. I pulled up her chest radiograph and stared at her lungs' new hazy white spots, a spring snowstorm. After nearly a century of beating, her heart was now newly skipping beats.

I worried about her. I knew we'd have to talk about death.

Standing in Mrs. B's curtained room, I wanted to ask her about her life, her loves, her values, and how she saw her future. I had a familiar urge to sit down next to her, to hold her hand, to give her time to let the questions, and sometimes the answers, sink in.

But COVID-19 preys on these comforts. Every moment I spend near my patients and every touch increases my chances of getting sick and potentially infecting others, too. Every day, I am pulling my end of a tug-of-war rope, trying to stay in the safe zone.

To stay safe, I have to build space and layer personal protective equipment between my patients and I—a yellow gown, a blue mask, white gloves, and a clear face shield. Only then can I cross the red line on the ground into their room—the hot zone. My patients are alone in the hot zone.

No visitors are allowed. At a stethoscope's length, I try to resist the urge to examine them too closely for long, limiting the time spent listening to the way air moves in and out of their lungs while I unconsciously hold my breath.

It is not lost on me that at a time when patients most require my presence and comfort, I am most constrained, and frankly scared, to give it. This virus is trying to teach me new ways of caring for them.

Talking to Mrs. B about life and death was never going to be easy, even before the pandemic. On that day, she couldn't hear me, her hearing aids forgotten on a counter at home. We got by with a mixture of loud single words—"pain?"—and miming symptoms. Exploring the intricacies of life and death in these improvised theatrics and with all this space between us seemed absurd at best, barbaric at worst.

In normal days, I wouldn't be wearing a mask—there is much we hear with our eyes and read with our lips. I would have gotten closer to her, crouched next to her good ear—which one was it?—and lowered the timbre of my voice to be heard. I learned that trick before the pandemic, watching family members translate my voice to an audible one. I thought of her family waiting at home and the solace they would give us both, in normal days, by being here. I didn't know how to give her the comfort of her doctor and of her daughter. It didn't feel fair to any of us.

They teach us how to comfort in medical school. It is both intuitive—the simplicity of a warm smile—and structured.

When I was in second year, they taught us how to have difficult conversations. I practised the skill with simulated patients with fake cancers and fake fathers who died, weighing my words and facial expressions carefully. I practised getting comfortable with the liminal silence that comes after shattering someone's world, realizing it never does get comfortable. I learned early on, from my first patient's death, the therapeutic value of touch, the comfort of holding a hand. "Cure sometimes, treat often, comfort always," said Hippocrates.

At a time when health-care workers like me are being lauded as superheroes, I worry that my patients are deprived of the simple power of comfort. In the past few months I have been wondering whether what I do is enough, whether my worry and my care are felt across the chasm of personal protective equipment, whether the tone of my voice and the choice of my words could sufficiently envelope them in my care.

The truth is, I have never felt so vulnerable, so aware that I, too, could catch this disease and become the patient. I try to think about what might give me comfort, beyond medical treatments, and I try to give them that, never sure if it's enough. The instinct to get closer to my patients tugs against my primal need for safety.

Mrs. B looked so small in her hospital bed. Like me in my PPE, she did not look like herself. Her short white hair was dishevelled from the ambulance gurney and the transfer to her hospital bed. Her sun patched hands rested on her belly, her wedding band loose on her thin finger. I held her hand and made a telephone sign with the other; I was going to call her daughter to give her an update and ask about any advance care directives. She squeezed my hand, not quite ready to let go. I held on a bit longer. She'd been alone so long.

I parted the curtains of her room, carefully weighing my decision to remove my layers of plastic armour. I wasn't sure how long I'd been in her room; time, like space, had transformed during the pandemic. It felt at once too short and too long.

"Don't you leave just yet."

I turned back around.

"How are *you* doing?" she asked me.

And in that moment, I knew she saw me as I was, a scared doctor doing her best, that maybe the tug-of-war rope I had been wrestling with was never meant to be pulled, but just held in each other's presence, a delicate bond between us. Maybe that was enough.

Note

1. "In the ER, Patients Need My Comfort but I Am Scared to Give It" was originally published in the *Globe and Mail*, June 5, 2020. Used with permission.

Vicissitude

PAM LENKOV

The patient's voice is changed. It is muffled and muted by the mask. But what is missing is so much more that might have been perceived—the indrawn breath that heralds a sensitive disclosure or a sob, or the split-second hesitancy of an open mouth before the words are uttered that has always made me consider the choice the patient made, what wasn't said but might have been in that brief managed time.

The mask is a hot gag that the patient and I are always aware of. It is a distraction when I want each word my patient says to be unencumbered, and I want my listening similarly to be. How can I concentrate when rivulets of sweat are coursing down my face in this claustrophobic antiviral housing, when I know the patient sees my discomposure?

The patient is alone. The website says visitors are not permitted. The signs at the entrance to the hospital say no visitors allowed but I know some have tried to plead in vain for the companion, who is ultimately relegated to waiting, even to participating by cellphone from the car.

What has been lost when the patient, unsupported, is young and moments away from receiving a cancer diagnosis? Much has been written about the fact that patients hear the *c* word and then not much else. I've learned to depend on the extra pair of ears, even if the friend or family member is as shocked at the hearing, and is trying to scribble or type details I am trying to parse in language free of jargon, while I know the patient is there but not there, suddenly having been thrust into a life forever altered, facing her mortality, and the terrifying limbo between diagnosis and what comes next.

But now I am alone with a patient who is alone, in a room smelling of disinfectant where a disembodied voice is asking question after question and I wear this PPE like a skin of helplessness.

The patient is sitting straight-backed and rigid in her chair while the voice probes relentlessly from the cellphone in her lap, her hands clenched around the armrests of the chair, as if the mask constrains not only her face but all movement. In her face all I can see are her pupils large and staring.

I see cancer in her eyes.

I miss the opportunity to observe. I miss the search for concordance between body language, demeanour, facial expression, and the patient's spoken words, that once, and perhaps unconsciously, identified allows a natural progression in the encounter, and the possibility of discordance that sets off my finely tuned antennae, alarm bells sounding a dissonance that I, like a detective, must try to tease out of my patient without disabling our engagement with each other. It is a powerful challenge and one I have been mourning these many weeks.

I miss the opportunity for the patient to observe me, for I can see my words, expressions, and demeanour mirrored in their responses. How can a patient navigate an interaction with a physician so encased, like some unwelcome apparition from a science fiction film?

I've suddenly become aware of my eyes, my eyebrows, how much of my forehead can be appreciated through the plastic. I've become so self-conscious of the modulation of my voice that I feel like an actor who's aware that an audition is going badly. No cadence, no volume, no syntax can soften those four words, "the biopsy showed cancer." I can't lean too far forward or sit alongside in the natural position of empathy previously taken with patients, especially when bearing bad news. I can't touch her shoulder. I'm hesitant to even proffer the box of tissue.

How can I deliver bad news when deprived of the tools to do so?

I teach medical students communication skills, taking and refining the particular gifts that helped them get this far and honing them into techniques and strategies that will allow them to successfully navigate future patient encounters.

I teach them how to convey empathy and explain that when a physician is truly empathic it allows us to put ourselves into a patient's shoes yet still enables us to maintain a distance that will facilitate a therapeutic agenda.

But I was never taught how to do this when I am so armoured against a viral pathogen that I feel robbed of the ability to express my humanity.

I feel inadequate to the task.

And I ask myself, if all is unchanged come September what will I, credibly, be able to teach them now?

I am struggling.

This is not the way I've taught students to practise medicine.

This is not the way I've practised medicine.

This is not the way I want to practise medicine, ever again.

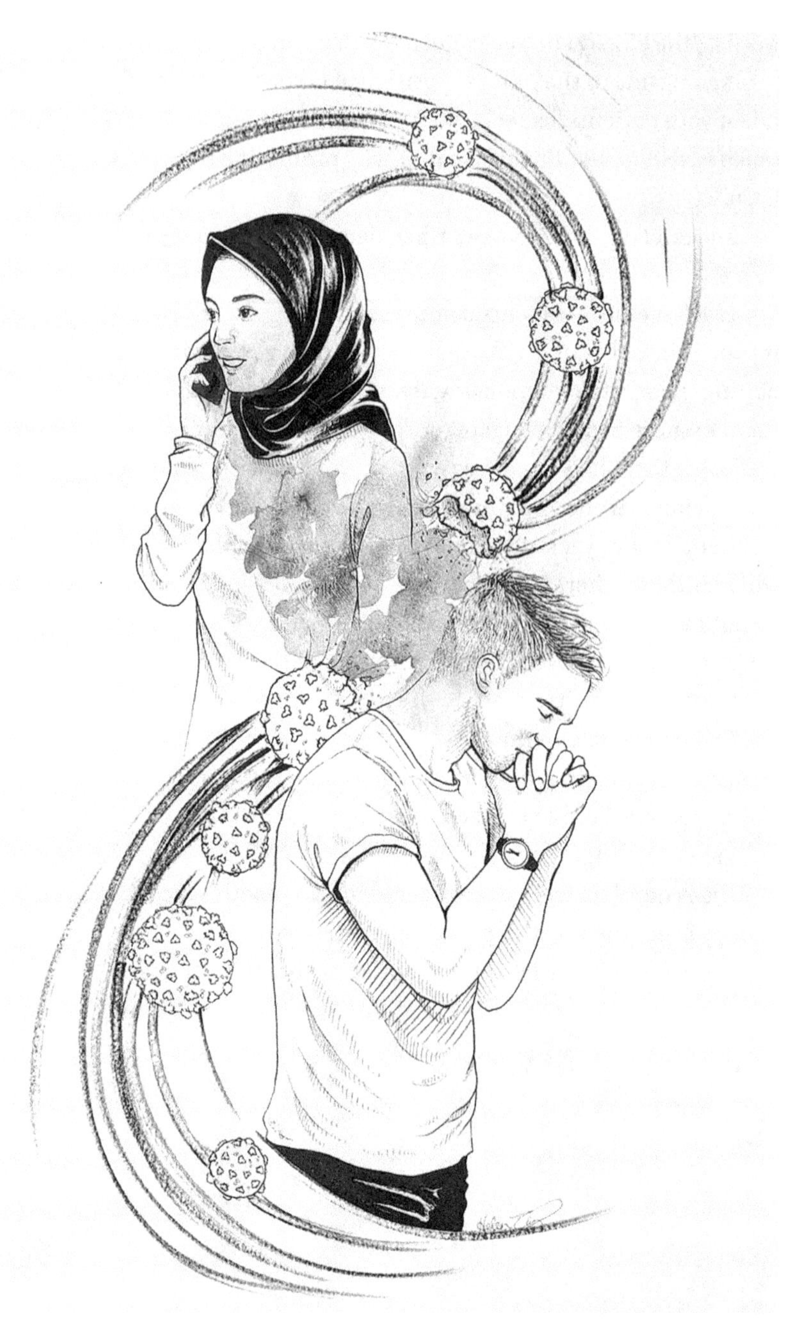

Connection by Helen Tang.

What Was Missing

MARGARET NOWACZYK

"Show me how you climb," I said to the little girl in my clinic room, one of identical twins, and patted the examining table. Sophie (*named changed*) was only the second patient I was seeing in person in our outpatient department since the beginning of the pandemic. It was the middle of August 2020, and our clinic—pediatric genetics and deemed non-essential—had been shut down since March 17, 2020. But this four-year-old girl needed abdominal ultrasounds and a measurement of the blood level for alpha-fetoprotein every three months; twice a year, she would come for a physical exam. All this, a part of tumour surveillance for Beckwith-Wiedemann syndrome, a genetic condition that carries with it an increased incidence of intrabdominal cancers. As is typical, Sophie's sister did not have the syndrome, an imprinting error that occurs during the twinning of a single fertilized egg.

The second-best way to make friends with a pediatric patient is to ask them to do something they are not allowed to do at home, like climb an examining table. The best? To ask them to jump while standing on the examining table, holding their hand, of course—a good neurological test for balance and co-ordination, in fact. As is climbing.

My little patient scaled the table with a hand from her mother and lay down on her back, her inquisitive little face intent on my masked one, her big blue eyes watching my every move. I lifted her tiny empire dress, frilled yellow with tiny flowers, and pressed on her belly, felt for masses, the Little Mermaid smiling at me from the front of her white undies.

I touched my hand to her warm skin. Her abdomen was soft, there was no tenderness on pressing down on her liver and spleen. "Everything's fine," I said and smoothed down the skirt of her dress, laid my hand flat over her belly. "We're done."

She stared at me and said, her voice sweet with that intense sincerity of a child: "Thank you, doctor."

I inhaled audibly. There was only so much that I could do not to hug her. Those unprompted words, so earnest, so real brought me close to tears.

I had missed being with patients so much.

The sister tugged at my dress. "Me too," she said not wanting to be left out, and, of course, I obliged. Sophie scooted away on the crinkling paper, and the twin climbed the examining table. I lifted the skirt of her identical yellow dress and pressed on her soft, warm abdomen. "Your tummy's fine, too," I said. She nodded sagely and slid off the table.

• • •

As a pediatric clinical geneticist, I have not seen a single patient with COVID during the entire pandemic. In March 2020, the disease spread out of China and wreaked havoc in Italy, the media choking with news of intensive care units and emergency departments overflowing with patients with pneumonitis and respiratory failure, of thousands of deaths among the elderly and the frail in Lombardy and Liguria. And Hamilton's McMaster Children's Hospital, where I work, was preparing for the worst. I—all of us—had no idea what to expect. Bodies in refrigerated trucks in hospital parking lots like in New York City? Terrified octogenarians dying in hospital hallways denied the sight of familiar faces, the touch of their son's or daughter's or grandchildren's hands? Respirator shortages? In short order, our hospital administration circulated an email questionnaire to all the physicians about what we would feel comfortable doing if we had to be redeployed.

Redeployed? Like in the army? My mind reeling with possibilities, each more dire, I ticked the box next to "Screening." I wasn't being flippant: the other choices—emergency room triage, hospital ward attending, or intensive care—were beyond my professional reach. I do not possess the skills to work in the emergency room or the intensive care unit; even a general pediatric ward would be a stretch. I wasn't afraid of COVID: I believed that with proper precautions and infection control I, a healthy fifty-six-year-old, would be safe. Asking people about their symptoms and contacts and travel history was the only thing I felt qualified to do. I have not started an intravenous line or prescribed medication since 1997. How could I care for critically sick patients when all I can do is examine bodies for genetically significant minor anomalies? For twenty-five years I have devoted my career solely to diagnosing genetic conditions in children and fetuses and to genetic counselling of adults. My skill set consisted of identifying and naming those tell-tale features and cohering them into recognizable syndromes, and ordering and interpreting the results of genetic tests. In the clinic, most of what I do is talk: explain complex genetic concepts in layperson's terms, inform the parents of the prognosis of their child's condition, or communicate bad news.

• • •

When the lockdown was announced in Ontario on March 13, 2020, all outpatient visits were cancelled. Our clinic manager began the task of reorganizing the clinic to see patients by video. The administrative staff, after having to cancel en masse all of our scheduled patients, were being certified to use the Ontario Telehealth Network and learning how to book online appointments. I was uneasy. I have never seen a patient that was not in the same physical space: so much is communicated by the way a mother tilts her head and cups her hand over her pregnant belly, by the way the father brushes the hair off his daughter's forehead, by the parents sitting together or apart. The technical/computer aspects were only a part of my worry. How would I tell a pregnant mother via a computer screen that her child had trisomy 18, a chromosomal anomaly that would render him mute and unresponsive and intellectually disabled? Or, worse, that we had no answer for the constellation of troubling black-and-white findings on the prenatal ultrasound? In the clinic, I reached out to touch my patients when they were upset, offered hugs if they seemed appropriate, or sat in silence—would my care and concern translate across the screen?

I had to consult on my first pandemic prenatal case even before I was certified to practice telemedicine, so the counselling had to happen by phone with the parents listening to me on their speakerphone. I spoke to them from my back deck on a hot June afternoon, the blossoming lindens of my neighbourhood scenting the air, so unlike the sterile atmosphere of the clinic room. I couldn't see the mother, I could only hear her voice—anxious and tense—and imagine how upset she must be. And even though it was a straightforward case, likely a normal baby with three tiny cysts studding the inner lining of the brain, I paced the deck like a caged lynx. After I reported the normal chromosomal results to the parents—trisomy 18 had been number one on the differential—they said they would continue the pregnancy. The whole time I felt like I was talking in the dark. I missed seeing the mother's eyes and face, seeing how she reacted in her body: tense shoulders? slumped back? All I had to go on was her intonations and the words she chose. "I wish I could have been there with you," I said at the end of the call.

Having been certified, I consulted on the next prenatal case by video: a fetus who initially was thought to have short limbs and a small chin. The mother had had an amniocentesis and this baby's chromosomes were also normal and, with the ultrasound images now showing normal growth, I could reassure her that things appeared to be on course. And it helped to see her without a mask covering the bottom of her face and to notice that she, too, had a small chin.

"Yes," she said when I mentioned it. "Until now, no physician has seen me without the mask on." Not being able to assess the facial features of the parents to determine if the baby's features were pathologic or familial became yet another casualty of the pandemic.

On another call, a couple booked for counselling about the recurrence risks of tuberous sclerosis kept their appointment only to tell us they'd had a miscarriage the day before. They were both crying and there was nothing I or the genetic counsellor could do but offer our condolences. In such a case, in person, I would have reached out, offered a hug. Locked in a screen, all I could do was say "I'm sorry" and watch their grief.

In time, it became a routine to "see" patients on my laptop in my sunroom, where the sun beat on my back through the skylights and the windows overlooked the maples, elm, and hemlock in the ravine below. Between the office assistants, genetics counsellors, and me, after a steep learning curve, we developed a workflow. Results and consult requests were scanned, encrypted, emailed to my inbox. And our patients were grateful for having access to genetic consultation and counselling despite the lockdown. Most patients were comfortable with the technology; many were genuinely grateful for not having to travel or visit a hospital and be exposed to COVID, and soon my misgivings dispersed.

And so it went. Summer 2020 arrived and some restrictions were lifted but we continued to see patients by telemedicine only. One day in mid-June, I sat in my hospital office, thoughts racing, unable to concentrate on anything, doom-scrolling COVID news. I was on call that week so I had filled out the online screening questionnaire, and, face masked and hands sanitized, presented my proof of negative screening to the security guard at the hospital entrance. That afternoon, my pager buzzed me out of the internet rabbit hole: the neonatal intensive care unit has just admitted a newborn with complex and unexpected anomalies. Excited to be needed, I climbed the stairs two at a time, stomped down the fourth-floor corridor, and scanned my ID at the unit's secure double door. At the nurses' desk, I asked where the new baby was. The receptionist looked at me askance and said that the baby was still in Labour & Delivery across the hall. I turned on my heel and dashed out. When the door to the resuscitation room whooshed open, five blue-masked faces turned toward me and I realized with horror that I didn't have mine on.

"Oh, shit," I said. "My mask! I just got up from my desk and ran when you called." I didn't want them to think that I was flouting the rules.

A nurse wordlessly pointed to the blue box with masks on the wall and I grabbed one.

"You got here faster than the surgeons," the neonatologist joked.

"Minus the mask, that is," I mumbled as I struggled to slip the ties behind my ears.

The speed with which I had run to see my first real live patient in weeks should have been a clue. All the technology, becoming proficient and efficient at electronic charting, improving my typing and retrieval skills, my whole techie evolution to catch up with the twenty-first century, had nothing on interacting with people: examining the baby under the warmth of the overhead heater, feeling the soft newborn skin under my fingertips, smelling that smell of freshly laundered hospital linens and a whiff of disinfectant. Discussing the findings with the neonatologist and neurosurgeon and the urologist, arriving at the most appropriate tests and management plan. Seeing the half-faces of my colleagues, eyes and bodies intent on giving the sick newborn the best care possible, and later, talking to the parents, seeing their eyes darting around the life support machinery, their bodies rigid. Having them all in my physical space—the examining room or the office—was what I was used to and that comfort was missing from the video calls. For a while, I didn't realize that something was missing—even seeing the newborn baby didn't drive the point home. It took another month of minimal human contact; it took Sophie and her twin sister, seeing her little face as she said, "thank you, doctor," hearing the soft, childish voice; being able to read her abdomen with my fingers in my clinic room five months after lockdown began, for the scales to fall off my eyes.

• • •

But something else was afoot, something I realized much later. With the outpatient clinic closed, with genetic care delivered by video, I must have subconsciously begun to worry whether I was superfluous. If the clinic could remain closed for five months without my seeing patients in real life, what did that say about genetic consultations? Definitely not an emergency, although in the prenatal clinic it could be. I felt useless, unneeded. All my training, all my experience—it seemed colleagues and patients were doing well enough without them. Was I even needed? Unnoticed, this gnawed on me, like a worm chewing underneath the skin of a seemingly healthy apple.

Beginning on November 1, 2020, McMaster Children's Hospital returned to pre-COVID patient volume, except that this time it combined in-person and virtual visits. But the first Monday was a hospital holiday that I had completely forgotten about—yet another day of isolation. The next day, two of my telemedicine patients cancelled. Unmoored, unoccupied, feeling painfully alone, I lumbered down two flights of stairs to the genetics outpatient clinic to find it deserted—only the receptionist and the genetic assistant sat sequestered in their plexiglass-delineated spaces, all of the five genetic counsellors working from home. I heard no voices, no kids zoomed around the waiting room, even the TV was turned off. All the surfaces in the examining rooms Viroxed, all the doors closed—a ghost clinic. My steps echoing in the empty hallway, I reeled with loneliness and returned to my office at an emotional nadir.

Wednesday, when I arrived for my awaited in-person clinic, I was delighted to find a resident waiting for me. Thankful for her company and interest, I taught her how to examine for arachnodactyly and increased arm span. I listed the Ghent diagnostic criteria for Marfan syndrome and the Beighton hypermobility score for Ehlers-Danlos syndrome, and the differences between the two conditions. I explained the different types of next-generation sequencing panels for both. The brown eyes above her mask smiled—she was engaged, enjoying our interaction. In the examining room, I got down on my hands and knees to assess a woman's heels for talus valgus. I joked with an eight-year-old about his fearsome *babcia* and told his mother that I, too, was raised by a Polish mother. The boy's parents and the resident laughed—I had told a joke, first in months. It helped that I diagnosed the boy with childhood-related hypermobility and not Ehlers-Danlos syndrome and that I was able to reassure his parents. It didn't matter that we all wore masks or that we couldn't shake hands—we were together.

Buzzed by the human contact and by the reciprocity of the social interactions, I happily plowed through a stack of charts, and read, edited, and electronically signed fifteen letters, but being in the land of the screens didn't bother me anymore. I chatted with the genetic counsellors—all five were in the office that day while until that day, for months, I had only seen them on Zoom calls for our semi-weekly meeting. I commiserated with the receptionist overwhelmed by a recent spate of rescheduled appointments in our office. I thanked the genetic assistant for the months of organizing the blood tests and send-outs for our video patients.

That afternoon, I had a standing Zoom call with a scientific program committee organizing the Canadian College of Medical Geneticists annual meeting—I was its chair. I knew that I had patients scheduled for the afternoon as well, but I thought those were video patients with the counsellors and I was planning to juggle them around my meeting. As I was slipping on my coat to rush home for lunch before the afternoon started, a counsellor asked me where I was going. "You have a combo clinic," she said. I stopped in my tracks. I haven't had a combo clinic since March. "Combo" clinics are those where a genetic counsellor interviews the patients and I examine them and, together, we propose a plan of testing and management. There were six such patients scheduled for that afternoon.

Normally, such a change in plans would have irritated me, but that day, my shoulders slid down my back and I smiled. I would work around my Zoom meeting and see the—actual, breathing, living—patients in the clinic. Ask them about their concerns and worries. Hear their inflection and diction and word choices. See their bodies react. Examine them for signs of genetic conditions—hypermobility of the joints, stretch marks, flat feet; listen to their hearts and lungs, and palpate their pulse on the inside of their wrists. Offer a diagnosis or reassurance or a plan genetic testing. I wriggled my arms out of my coat, hung it on the door, and walked down the corridor to the clinic room. I knocked on the door and slipped inside.

"Hi, I'm Dr. Nowaczyk," I said to the middle-aged woman sitting on the examining table. "It's so nice to meet you."

A Family History in 2 Pandemics, 4 Infections, and 102 Years

JILLIAN HORTON

My great-grandmother died in 1918. She's buried a few miles from my home, in a cemetery where stones are periodically vandalized. She eluded Russian pogroms only to succumb, at thirty-two, to the Spanish flu, leaving two small girls motherless. That's most of what I know about her: the hole she left. The long, shifting shadow of her death, its fingers still reaching out occasionally to tap the shoulder of descendants in this generation, now in the midst of our own pandemic.

My grandmother, Yetta, lived and died in that shadow. The mother who vanished when she was just two years old could never be made to reappear, and so her older sister rose to the occasion. That was even the sister's name: Rose. But a few years later, their father married a woman who saw Yetta as the spectre of the dead, revered wife, a bright spot she could never scrub from her husband's memory. The stepmother made it clear: Yetta's father was not to show Yetta love. Love belonged to *her*. If he wanted to give Yetta so much as a worthless trinket, a pitiful homage to the life they'd led before the pandemic destroyed it, it had to be smuggled through Rose. Love shrivelled up like a raisin in that home, was never an option again.

It was no surprise, really, that when my grandmother met my grandfather at seventeen, she leapt impulsively at the chance for a new life. They had a baby in their first few years of marriage. When he was two, he died suddenly, from yet another kind of infection. My mother would never have known about him except one day, when she was a little girl, she unearthed a cardboard box under her parents' bed. Papers with an unfamiliar name on them, a few black-and-white pictures, booties. Proof of a life. She somehow knew not to ask about this phantom boy, knew even at that age she had unearthed an unspeakable, timeless hurt.

Sometimes I imagine my grandmother, carrying those shadow losses with her. Their interminable weight. A crushing, stifling grief, the kind that takes your breath away, makes your heart crack pitifully, like the shell of an egg. A grief dating back to 1918, one that made my grandmother retreat into herself, made her raise *my* mother with a fixed gaze and a sharp tongue. Hardening, then hardening further, until she was petrified.

"She never had a kind word to say," my mother told me once. "It was as if she didn't even know how to say those words."

I wonder what it was like for Yetta, to lose her mother. The shipwreck of the life she might have known, invisible injuries that lasted her whole life. My own mother was exasperated by Yetta's deficiencies but also beholden to her, making the pilgrimage out to her home on the West Coast, always bearing offerings—purses, books, scarves, all laid at the altar of Yetta's feet—as if this would be the time when Yetta would finally bestow her approval. But my mother never got the nod of her mother's unconditional love—because Yetta was never capable of *giving* it. Because Yetta never had it *herself.* Because it died, with her mother, in the 1918 epidemic, a loss she—and her descendants—would feel for over a hundred years.

My aunt made a series of tapes once. Interviews with Yetta, near the end of her life, unburdening herself. One day, when the tape recorder was off, Yetta said to my aunt, "I know why I'm the way I am. But what I didn't realize is how much it affected other people."

I wonder if what she really meant was that she *infected* other people.

Maybe that's why this spring, as this great pandemic began to upend my life, I realized with some surprise: the last one affected me too. I began to think of my genealogy by microbe, starting with my great-grandmother. Then my shoebox uncle, dead in babyhood, almost certainly from an illness for which there is now a vaccine or medicine. Then, later, the loss of my own sister, after a long and brutal decline set off by the scourge of patients on antibiotics, C. Difficile. And most recently, my brother, who lived with a series of health issues that began with in utero German measles, acquired only months before the life-saving vaccine became available. He died of pneumonia during *this* pandemic, one more name in the lineage of suffering. Or maybe one more, for now.

I always had a feeling, growing up, that my family's life had been kicked in by an unseen force, upended, seeded with an indescribable sadness. I didn't know that this story was *the* story. Not the story of our lives, but the story of life on *Earth*—the one where we have to coexist as best we can with organisms that have always kicked over the things we hold most sacred. What do they leave in their wake? Newspaper clippings in a box under a bed, names written mournfully in stone, yellowed photographs on living room walls. Proof that we are not invincible, that the things we love can be quickly upended by improbable, invisible vandals.

Now, in homage to Yetta, to her losses, to *my* losses, to history's endless loop, I isolate at home, and send my mother offerings. Hand sanitizer. Lysol wipes, bleach spray. Masking always, trying not to infect the next generation with the consequences of my choices. And trying to outwit a hundred-year-old grief while I wait to move out of its shadow, back into the light.

Endurance

MANISHA BHARADIA

"Drop me at Walmart," she says, "Or better yet, just drop me here."

"We're on McLeod Trail, Ba. I'm not going to drop you on the side of the road."

"You have to do your thing. Drop me here so I can have some freedom! I haven't been able to do anything since this COVID thing." She exclaims this, cleverly, using the outburst as justification to remove her mask. The outrageous clashing blue mask. The restrictive paper havoc. Blocker of smiles and laughs.

"This is too much," she says.

Yet again, I remind her, as gently as possible, "Ba, you have to wear your mask. I should already be doing your groceries for you. But, since you are here, you have to. It's a 'rule.'"

"Rules" take on a more suggestive character for a Gujarati woman in her late seventies. A woman who cooked three meals a day for a family of thirteen, after relocating to another continent, after being married to a stranger, all before her seventeenth birthday.

"Rules"

The futility of this word seals us inside the bubble that is my Nissan Juke. Sunday adventure drive becomes sterile void.

Maybe it was inevitable. 2020—the year of enclosure. Bubbles inside of bubbles. Trying (but failing) to tame (and restrain) this powerhouse of a woman.

A woman who has endured.

A woman who is beginning to recognize just how much enduring has been done in the seventy-six years of her life.

So, I can see how she views adversity as a curious jester—no real threat. She has made it this far—the seventy-six years culminated into a fortress of goodwill and Brahma Kumaris.

So, I know when I say "rules" she thinks "watch me." And while nothing gives me more life than to see her raw vivacity, nothing terrorizes me more than a microscopic particle entering her upper airway. Her beautiful nose or mouth.

Causing her, yet again, to endure.

Blowing Smoke in Your Ear

ANDREW HOWE, ANGELA E. SIMMONDS, BOBBY TAYLOR, and DOLLY WILLIAMS; facilitated by ARUNDHATI DHARA and CHADWICK WILLIAMS

In the spring of 2020, when COVID-19 was new and raging and everyone went home and locked their doors, the African Nova Scotian (ANS) community experienced an outbreak of coronavirus. There were many media accounts of what occurred, but very little about living through the first wave of COVID-19 from the community itself. What follows is the result of conversations with community leaders who consented to a project without a clear form, but with a clear question: What does care and health mean to the ANS community in the face of a global pandemic?

This was never constructed as a research project. Rather, it is the result of generous introductions and the sharing of knowledge by people in Cherry Brook and the Preston communities. In other times, I was told these conversations would be had at kitchen tables over a meal, but the ongoing pandemic made that impossible. In fact, kitchen table conversation is a specific form of community engagement that asks people to speak in small groups, often with questions to guide discussions. While this project was always meant to be literary and narrative in nature, these reflections draw from that tradition.

The result is a careful curation of the ideas and stories that the participants so generously shared about their experiences and the resilience of their communities. There has been editing for syntax and clarity, but the ideas are theirs. Each participant has reviewed the manuscript and has been able to ensure that their words and meaning have not been misrepresented. We acknowledge that the process of curation is not without perspective, and as health-care providers we bring yet more of ourselves to this project. We are especially grateful for the direction of the participants in getting their stories right.

• • •

BOBBY: I remember my grandmother when I was kid, I used to go to her place. And that's where she made medicine. All of the stuff that she used was stuff that grows in the yard right now: dandelion root and spruce bark and these little pine needles and these little berries and just all of these random things that are in the yard that she knew.

I had a cold. I was like, there's no way I'm drinking that.

It was my grandmother.

I drank it.

She says, drink that—you drink it, drink it, and you feel better. It was disgusting, but it was one of those things. My grandmother's medicines.

I was doing some research the other day looking into dandelion roots and how good it is for you and how it helps with your heart and all of these other things, and I found out that the same company that makes heart medication makes Roundup.

ANDREW: The African Nova Scotians were [here] from the very beginning. There is no Nova Scotia history with[out] the African Nova Scotians. The easiest way to reconcile that is to think about that term that I'm using—*African Nova Scotian.* You're not going to hear that anywhere else in Canada.

There's no African Ontarian—that just doesn't exist. But because of the history here in Nova Scotia with Black loyalists, Jamaican Maroons, and Black refugees from the mid-1700s, before there was Canada, [there] were African Nova Scotians.

That alone should highlight the importance of the community...the value and the contributions that our community has brought to Nova Scotia and to Canada as a whole.

ANGELA: And I say this with all caveats of community spirit, but the reality is that [they are] very oppressed communit[ies]. That's the narrative that I want to change. There's a real difference [in] the way society sees East Preston, North Preston, Cherry Brook. There is [also] a narrative of a future, of pride.

Even within the communities, there's a divide that we just need to work past. It used to be [called], Preston Township in a way that Black communities [could] come together.

• • •

BOBBY: Everything you hear about us comes from people who have studied up, or they've done a research project, or they've done a pilot project and then they take those results and they say for us, health care is done.

DOLLY: It's a very resilient community, East Preston, we go out and we help each other.

ANDREW: It's a small tight-knit community with historic roots, historic families. And it's a place where people try to live their lives just like everybody else does without all of the extra barriers that are in place. From directly in the law to just in people's prejudices and everywhere in between, [as] if those didn't exist.

They all want to have a place where they can live and raise their families.

Basically [they] just asked me to help getting stuff started down here. And I just said, well, [I'm] sitting around the house, not doing anything. I mean, it's the least you can do, right?

BOBBY: The importance of this community [is] we have a huge, great history in this place. We have history right here before Canada was a country. Some of us are refugees from the War of 1812, you know? Some of us actually had a hand in building [this place]. It's not like we're just tagalongs to the priority. You know, we actually had a lot to do with [the history of this] province and to be treated the way we were treated [by] government and the health-care system is ridiculous.

The fact that if I had a heart attack at my house, I'm going to die before I get to a hospital? You know what I mean? If I had a stroke, chances are by the time I get to the hospital, it's going to be irreversible. You know, when you live like that, what does health care really matter?

DOLLY: In my community, the problem was the health-care system [not] coming with a priority even when there *was* COVID.

• • •

ANDREW: It's like, government thought they could call out North Preston for having people not following the rules, but other [communities], white communities, are doing this all at the same time and nobody really knew what was actually going on at the beginning of the pandemic.[1]

People would've been mad about that. And rightfully so.

BOBBY: Anything that happens in the Black community gets put on blast, like it's the worst thing in the world. They [say], "Look at these people over here doing this and doing that and look how they're living, blah, blah, blah."

ANGELA: [It was] on TV. I remember very clearly hearing that and thinking, oh my gosh, I'm so embarrassed. [But] I shouldn't have been, right? I was just like, oh my gosh, but I could work from home. So at that point, it wasn't even about trying to go into work and try to figure [out what to say to people]. But it was embarrassing and then you were angry.

ANDREW: And then their unwillingness to simply admit that they were wrong for doing it. That reinforces a pretty damaging and one-dimensional vision of what it means to live and be in the Prestons and Cherry Brook.

DOLLY: A lot of negativity went on. People have this, yes, people in the community had COVID. But the people in the community that had COVID took care of themselves, but also those who didn't have COVID went to help those people.

People need to understand what respect is. And what faith is and giving back to community is. If I want the respect myself, and I want you to [be] better, well, I have to respect my neighbour and their children.

ANDREW: When all of that stuff was going on it would reinforce the mistrust of the public health system. Because they're ready to just throw you under the bus. Then you turn around and you see all these other people from all across the province talking about, oh, well, there they go again causing trouble for everybody.

It was a long time and a long conversation to get them to admit that they were wrong for doing that. As far as I can remember, they never did actually say that. But they tried to rectify it later on. How effective that was is up to debate.

That kind of stuff happens and the long-term effect of it is stigma that permeates through Nova Scotia. If they say, "I saw somebody from the community," when you see that mentioned somewhere, they're talking about all Black people in Nova Scotia, it's really code for the dark-skin people.

And that's the type of thing that the community had to deal with on top of this virus that nobody knew nothing about, but they knew that it was killing people.

DOLLY: Yeah, the health care wasn't here, but they said that it was [many] communities...[not] just this community.

And yet they named the Prestons—always, we always [got] to be on the news—but if something comes up negative about our community, okay, let's right [it]. Fix it.

People say I'm different, but I have a lot of respect for doctors.

ANGELA: There was that anger; how dare you call us [out]? Once again, our blackness is now negative. It's not just about community. It's about who we are, how we show up in this society, how we contribute. And once again we don't contribute in a positive way. And now you're telling us that all that we have done has been nothing because now we're carrying the disease. Which [at that time made people feel] ashamed. Like you didn't even want to get tested, you didn't want to do anything. No one wanted to get tested because no one wanted to know.

BOBBY: We have an outbreak and you're not going to treat us? You're not going to help us? What does that say about us? Just as people, do you even see us as people? Because you don't do stuff like that [in] all these other places [with outbreaks].

ANGELA: And in the community, there was a beginning of a divide. [People were] getting upset when more than one person went into a grocery store or started listening and thinking, Oh was it so-and-so that brought it here? And so that initial response to be angry then turned into [a] divided community. Which is what people do in communities that have been oppressed. Because we couldn't support one another in a way that could address community.

BOBBY: Fear mongering doesn't work in the Black view, and the biggest thing now is to have government look at the Black community and say, You need to trust us.

They'll tell you one thing and yeah, you'll get that one thing, but they don't tell you everything. They don't tell you the control that they're going to have over you because of it.

• • •

DOLLY: I didn't get upset. I said, well, I'm glad to know. We know it's here. Let's do something about it. It's here, but it's not only the Black community.

Oh, good. I know what's going on. I can get my stuff together [and] let my family know that COVID is in East Preston. So what are we going to do?

I took it and spun it around that I can use this for my benefit. To help me and my family and also call the seniors and say COVID is in the community. I took it and use it.

ANGELA: It's women. It's young girls, our elders, that's who takes the leadership in community [and] who does care in particular. Probably for the harder tasks, [the] labour [of] health and care and how you show up I think men would take a role, but definitely not in the same way [as] women. It's not a burden, but it is the oldest daughter, and then the youngest child, so it's always rolled down into women and young women. It's a piece they hold for [us]. It's good and bad, but [it is what it is].

ANDREW: I guess this is all hindsight now, but what would have happened if that initial group [of community organizations] had not pushed for testing in the community and getting resources to the community as they were needed? What would have happened or what could have happened if they hadn't done that? Would the department of health have been thinking about that?

I don't think so. And so we could have been in a very different situation, had the community not stepped up to take care of themselves at the very beginning. I mean, once we got established, then health was there and they wanted testing and this and that and [they wanted it] every five minutes. But [what] if that had not initially happened, if the community had not initially pushed back? When they were ostracized...then where would we be now? Thinking about that is a conversation for health to have and for health to think about. Would we have done the right things?

Really think about it, though. Really think about it. Would [they] have, would you have really? That's something that I think could be a conversation. Later on, but it's not something that should be forgotten. I mean, I'm only one person, but it's certainly not something that will be forgotten anytime soon.

DOLLY: I think that the health department was weak, regardless. They brought out the vans and all that, [the one that] gives the [tests] afterwards. But it had to be asked for. All those things that happened shouldn't have to be asked [for]. It should be automatic. We have a health office downtown, but that place should be flourishing.

BOBBY: I know this has nothing to do with COVID, but they're using the whole COVID shutdown to do all their stuff because we can't meet [in] public. Can't talk about it. We can't protest it. We can't do these things. And they're doing all of these things and we have no stakes because the law says we can't get out there amongst each other.

You need to prove yourself. Your words are always mixed.

I'm the chair of a community organizing [group]. And I was getting phone calls from people saying they went to the hospital and once they swiped their health card and their postal code came up [and it] was flagged as an outbreak [area]. They basically said they couldn't treat them.

And I said, one you're already there. So [if] anything is going to happen. It's already happening. And two, what business do [they] have telling me that [they] can't treat me when I paid for [it with taxes]?

I was done with the whole thing. How are you going to say there's a pandemic in the province?

It's not like we're just making this stuff up. It's a real thing. They stopped treating us in the hospital. Like our COVID is different from everybody else.

• • •

DOLLY: It was like a pain when I couldn't visit. Personal hugs, personal touch, personal family, caring. I get to see some people now. I'm one of the fortunate ones that can get out. But I say for a lot of the people in the community...they don't have that option. They wait for someone to get them.

ANDREW: One of the things—I don't know if it was done properly or not—[no], I won't say properly. It could have been a bigger focus would have been people's mental health. That was one of the major concerns with the community. The Black community here in Nova Scotia, and I'm sure beyond, are very social—just the community structure and design [of] the community. It really depends on other people in the community. And so of course being isolated from them, not being able to see family...

ANGELA: All of a sudden [we see the news conferences] but [they're] really not understanding that people have a different way of speaking, [of living]. In communities saying you have a bubble of family in your house, while most times the house is ten people or the neighbour beside us is our family? So you're not going to tell me I can't go next door to see my daughter.

[And] sometimes the grandmother *is* the mother, that other mother figure [a child] needs to be [there]. And well, my grandson is coming. I don't know what everyone else is talking about, but I'm telling my grandson you're coming up. And that really is what happened. There was a reality that you're not going to tell me I can't see my family. So to hear [that] we may have to pick and choose? Well, that's not happening in our community.

BOBBY: And that's the strength for our community—just being together, communal living. We go to church together. We go to the grandmother's house on Sunday [with]...the whole family—and we have big families.

You know, I can't talk to anybody in my family.

I have a wife and two kids, you know what I mean? So that's what I do. I pick my mother over my aunt or my uncle, do I pick my brother or my sister? If you're following these rules, you can't actually have a real family or a real community. That's the problem because that's how we've survived here this whole time.

• • •

ANDREW: We can't go to work because we're isolating. So what are we going to do? Taking care of that type of thing was a big part of care.

ANGELA: When [they] were saying only go to the store every two weeks, and then when it came to the point of only being able to use debit, like what [about] people [who use] cash? [I have had] days of just having cash and counting down, because when you're banking money you account for [when it's gone]. So you literally [get cash] before the bills go. There's no way I could have wait[ed]. Like I [can't be] waiting to go to the grocery store [every two weeks].

DOLLY: I work at a shelter. We had people come in and we put them in an isolation room for a bit.

I worried even there [for] my community. I worried about the homeless people. What's going to happen to those on the street, what's going to happen? Those homeless people that got no place to go, where are they gonna go? They got no place. They on the street, I go into the city [and] they're sitting on a bench at night.

Well, Lord, you know, these people got no place to go. I pray that [they] get better services. That's one thing that COVID brought out; the racism, the poverty levels, the sexism, all the isms, that those are ways within government and within a community that we don't talk about.

ANGELA: So I was very frustrated [because] there was just such an enormous amount of privilege that was coming with all of this information. And that made me a bit more angry and a bit more resistant to even listen. [But in the end], I was going to take care of my health and definitely do what I had to do to keep our family safe and community safe. But at the same time, I lost a lot of respect for authority and how we go about following the rules that were set on us that didn't consider us when they were being made.

DOLLY: And if there wasn't a family member there, they would call somebody else in the community. Can you come and pick up stuff?

ANGELA: I started working from home. And I would say that one of the biggest struggles that I think about is not getting the support from work in terms of understanding [the situation]. When seniors didn't have access to food and [we] wanted to drop food off and then explaining that to an employer? It was difficult. I literally had to take vacation. They didn't understand the dynamics of my pastor calling to say, Can we get the truck? Or someone from community saying we have ten bags of groceries, [and] we don't have a vehicle. Can you come up and [help]? Like, those were things that happened. It was work, 'cause we were [all] trying to survive.

• • •

ANDREW: The churches in the three communities are of course the centre of them.

DOLLY: You know what? I have this family, I forget the name of the church, but it's not from here. The minister showed up at my door with lunch fully prepared. I wasn't expecting it.

I said, I'm good.

"No, that's okay. We're doing it. And you're part of this."

What a blessing. People care, other people care.

The community going and taking care of people, making sure they got what they need to do and go pick up the groceries, go get the medicine, do the things they need to do.

ANDREW: Calling on the church members to help with deliveries, being able to use them as a resource. But also them being able to shift their worship online. Being able to still connect with community members who wouldn't have been online. So that not only could we continue to share information about what was going on in the community, but also being able to [have] fellowship with each other as well.

DOLLY: I went one day and wanted to go down to the doctor. I couldn't get into the building. Won't even let me in. You can't come in. If you're isolated you should get a walk in and talk to somebody. But I just found that those kinds of situations, people are afraid that you're going to bring something to them.

ANDREW: That was one of the most important things for the church, so that they could maintain that connection with people. Something as simple as bringing back the old school—I don't even know what they call them—but you call somebody, you pray with them and then they call somebody else and then they pray with them.

DOLLY: That part [was what] I missed the most—not being able to go to church and hear the choir, get up there and rock with the church and do my thing. Instead [it was] me at my house and doing it, and it was like, I'm here, but it's not the same thing. But, you got to get this [COVID] cleared up.

ANGELA: What COVID has shown us is that there's different ways of praying. There's different ways of having spiritual relationships with God. I think one of the things that our church, in particular in this community, has to do is learn to adapt and grow with that. And in order to continue the spirit of the churches in community, we have to embrace differently what prayer looks like for folks. At the end of the day there's no greater comfort than sitting in church and feeling the presence of God and that spirit come to you.

• • •

DOLLY: I guess I just find that the fear is there. But like I said, I been tested so many times.

ANDREW: The fear of, I guess, the fear of the unknowing. Not knowing fully what, what the disease was. Nobody knew of course, not just people in the community. We didn't know what it was.

All we knew was that it was contagious and it was bad. So that would have brought a lot of fear...where you would have your immediate family...take care of whatever you needed.

If I had got COVID and was laid up, I wouldn't be calling some of the people that I would call up for some other stuff. Any other day type of thing. Because, like I said, we don't know. We didn't know what it was. I wouldn't want them to come over here and then it ends up over there.

DOLLY: [If] someone comes to your funeral and takes that disease to your family? [I'd] rather be healthy and [have] a family to be able to come back [to] and visit [when I'm] right.

• • •

DOLLY: I have to say that back in the days, the older people had had less knowledge, but they had more common sense. They did more with little, we have more and [are] doing less. When something happens, it's always blame this one or blame that one. But what about looking in the mirror and seeing what am I doing to make it [right]?

And that's the way I look [at it] when someone says to me, I'm not getting the needle. Well, that's your right. But you're affecting me and other people. So I'm going to tell you how I feel. You might not want to hear it.

So I could call people and they went in and got the shots.

BOBBY: At the same time, we're a God-fearing people, so we're very comfortable putting it in God. Like I tell people all the time, I'm not afraid of COVID. It is what it is, you're not going to be able to control it.

DOLLY: I've got my shots. I'm not saying I'm not going to get sick. But I am saying that I believe that God is my strength. And that we believe with the faith, that God is in charge of everything.

Don't make me feel bad. I got the needle—respect my right to get the needle. And the fact that my family has all got their needles and my grandkids can't get the needle saying, well, when can I get it?

BOBBY: But if you have a question about it, you're labelled anti-vaccine and then people would just lambaste you. I think the vaccine would be a great thing. If it works, get the vaccine. But I don't forget everything that set [us] up, you know?

And when it first came out, [COVID] was like the flu. If you're sick or you have health conditions...that could be exacerbated. But everybody else you ride it out and then [in] two weeks you'll be fine.

And that's the way a lot of people[are] thinking, I mean, this is not just a Black [thing, it's] a worldwide thing. And if I get sick and I stay home for two weeks and I'll be fine, then what's the thing with getting the vaccine?

DOLLY: I get upset when people say, well, I'm not going to do it.

It's not a right. You infringed on my right when you disrespect me. And you'll say you're not going to get the vaccine, but you want to walk around into community and do whatever you want.

That's a disrespect of every one of us, because the signs are telling us that we need the vaccine and that's going to protect us.

[If I] go up there without my mask and not washing my hands and doing all those things, I'm putting other people in jeopardy without even knowing it, like not conscious of what [I'm] doing. [There is] a lack of education in the health-care system within our communities.

It could have been a lot worse. Even though they got the needles, you still hear them saying them saying "I only got it because I got [sick]."

One of the girls said, "Well, I'm a Christian, I'm [not] going to get sick." I said, "Yeah, you're a Christian, I'm a Christian too, but God gave me common sense." He also gave the doctors and the scientists and knowledge to make these things available to us. When did you ever see people in Nova Scotia march against health care? They're there to protect you and to help. Wait a minute, pull yourself back and look at what you're doing.

Because when you say well, we don't want this, you're not only blocking the people that want it, but you're damaging the whole community.

BOBBY: Technically it is [a] right. But [that's only] one way of thinking. There's one way of looking at it and anybody who doesn't look it at that way is lazy. Add that [to the] discrimination in our community—you know, we already have enough stigma.

We already have strikes against us.

This vaccine is just another. And with the way they treated us the last time [during the first wave of the pandemic], it's like, [if we don't] as a whole entire community [bow] down and get this vaccine, are they just going to block our community off?

Is that how it's going to go? Because you pretty much did that the last time.

So many people treat the vaccine like it's a cure. And I'm like, well, maybe so. But what they told you was that the trial, when they first started, they said they don't know [what was] going to happen.

They think this is the best option. But for me in dealing with *this* health care, that's not good enough, and for a lot of [other] people, that's not good enough. I don't really want to fix anything for your test.

• • •

ANDREW: There was a lot of community building in that way that was able to continue. I noticed a lot of people and groups who don't usually work together were making a special effort to work together to get things done. Working with the daycares and the rec centres, the halls, the auxiliary groups that are throughout the community, being able to pull them all together during that time to make sure that there was a large reach in the community.

DOLLY: Young people from the community, they were going out and bagging vegetables and stuff and bringing it to people's homes, especially seniors. And they started up [from] the get-go. But they do that anyway, every year [they] bring [this] to the community, by the back door, behind the scenes. And I love them. In fact, they doing stuff all the time. They're having bake sales to raise money, to do things for others. They give back to the community. I should say [the food bank] started sending bags of groceries. One that come and I said, "What's that doing [on] my step?" But it didn't matter whether you used a food bank or didn't use a food bank. They went across the board, they delivered door to door. Whether they know you [need food] or not, they delivered. So for me, that was a program that was non-discriminatory. They took care. They were taking care of everybody and that's the way society should be.

BOBBY: For us, health care takes place in our community. If a Black person goes to the hospital, more often than not, they think they're going to die. And that's why they'll do *anything* else. They'll say, yeah, whatever I just ride.

ANGELA: Health and caring in community looks so much better than when you go to the doctor. Even in our own history—you know, I remember growing up and when I had an earache my dad blowing smoke from the pipe in your ear to be like, it's okay. [Or] when my kids had the hiccups, we'd put a cross with toothpicks on their forehead to get rid of hiccups. Then you go to [the doctor and] sometimes there's ointments that you can be putting on your forehead to take away headaches, you know?

Care is being able to show up and listen to someone and really be kind and gentle. You know, I hate to say, [but] the [hospital is] not a care place for me. The way in which we're greeted at the doors, [not] understanding how folks are in trauma, in their own self and in a busy kind of environment dealing with so many things.

BOBBY: That's health care for us. That's what it is, what it's always been.

• • •

DOLLY: It shouldn't be because COVID comes. Somebody's got to get up and take care of my brother and sister for me again. I got a Bible says, take care of your neighbours. My neighbour doesn't mean my neighbours. It means my people, my community as a whole.

When we have a meeting in our community, pay attention to the issues going on. Don't just stand there and complain. They saw what COVID did, they saw what happened. And you can make a change with your voice. Don't sit home and talk about it. I'm hoping that when this is all over, those people will come out and be a part of the solution [because we] have to get that problem solved.

I see this community as coming closer, I'm hoping that we're going to become closer and drawn closer [together]. [So] when something happens, [we] come together and work together as a team and build that relationship for our community.

ANGELA: No one ever wants to hear the story, to really dig in and ask the questions. When [people] hear the same voices with the same narrative, there's this idea that [they] *know*. [But] it doesn't fly anymore, it doesn't matter.

ANDREW: ...Unlearn what you thought. That's the easiest way to put it. And when you think about...what is East Preston? What is North Preston? What [is] Cherry Brook?

What you thought you heard about it or what you thought you knew about it? That's not going to be the whole story or it might not even be part of the story.

Note

1. In April 2020 Preston Township communities were singled out by name as COVID hotspots in a televised press conference. Then Premier Stephen McNeil suggested that members of the communities were "reckless" and would not "stop partying," leading to the spread of the virus. During the same press conference, Nova Scotia's first COVID death was announced.

It's Hard Not to Slam a Fist on the Table When the Finish Line Keeps Lurching Further Ahead, or Third Wave

CANDACE DE TAEYE

Maybe you were a mother...
Maybe you were dead. There are ways
to be both.

—SHIRA ERLICHMAN, "Odes to Lithium"

no Sir, take a moment to say goodbye to your mother you understand there are only two absolutely no visitors outcome in hospital I'll be in the hall take a minute please he's mastered mute unmute and refreshing the page at six years old family quarantine round three no tail end of lounge wear or feral toddler sussing out the cupboards badly hidden wrappers in the

couch   damn sneaky raccoons   days of screen time   dubious
exposure   the man   screened   negative   eye protection   only
required   for failed   screenings   goggles overtop prescription
glasses always fogging   rivulets looks silence despondence   en
route the trauma centre one drink too many step ladder slipped
affixing   failed is insensitive   the noose   a positive   household
contact   noted in the sending documents   I had secured   his
stretcher straps   just prior   I had secured concert tickets   no   a
vaccine appointment   for the next day   it had only taken   three
hours   of constant   refreshing   on my phone screen   I had to
cancel   and isolate   teach   the six-year-old   still life practice
in pastels   call my dad   the most self-aware   alcoholism   I'm
worried about   his   isolation   despite the bodies   filling up
refrigerated transport trucks   in the forest city   he's full of guilt
grown of absence   my learned   foresight   to buy a couple   extra
presence   for my kids   write his name   he listens   hesitates   to
disclose much   some weeks   but always calls   often asks   how I'm
getting along   with my spouse   confesses to him   my husband
that is   one night over drinks   how he regrets leaving my mom
my mom   hesitates   about   the vaccine   despite   working in a
hospital   and chronic bronchitis   grade one teacher   scolds
intermittently   through floorboards   the youngest child   finally
into outdoor preschool   this is   respite care   two days a week
they tried   to skip over us   because   my job   a perceived risk   to
the cohort   I called them   out on it   I need this   he comes home
smelling   of homemade   beef barley soup   paints with beet juice
North American doctors   may soon   make decisions   based on
resource scarcity   now let us introduce   the term   moral injury
your cake   is illegal   the co-worker hissed   get fucked   so is the
twelve of us   in this room   using common dishes   hand washed
in Dawn   double-think is   essential work   this other woman is
ninety-six years old   speaks only Russian   what would you do?
her family asks   there are   no visitors   my chorus refrain   a
chance   she could die   at home   surrounded by family   or   she
can come with us   to hospital   a year ago   there would have been
no question   on their part   the full toll   would consider   the

backlog of surgeries imaging those who will certainly die of
previously treatable also so many seniors too afraid to call
us disease vectors to our faces to invite us over their
threshold too afraid of the hospital right now choosing
death instead of stents this woman had the most advanced
breast cancer I've ever hard purple bleeding orange peel how
big was it first lockdown ? a thumbnail she stays invites her
family for Easter next Sunday it's still much too soon to
consider the pandemic positively impacting our concept of
death care not framed as medical failure palliation at home
the idea of a good death is an essay I've been trying to write
forever but I sleep a lot now maybe too much on spouse's
birthday after I shuck a few bivalves make elaborate
quarantinis we argue intensely I catch a glimpse of terror
desperation I've not seen before now realize he needs
reassurance is not unworthy of love despite adulterous past
lovers a complicated backstory with his mother depression
I have never understood women who choose a man over
their children he cannot comprehend out-sourcing physical
affection or sex despite my offering up a hall pass he's a
monogamist at heart which isn't a bad thing but you should
anticipate drought conditions with young children years of
working opposites I am acutely out of my body no visitors
please I have been the eldest son states the worst part about
this family is that we are all heartbroken September is
coming they'll both be in school will it be easier then? I believe
in quieter should be cherishing this time I'm told they grow
so fast the crafts and costumes epoch of the pandemic ended
months ago children are an indicator species of a community
did you know biologists have observed that urban squirrels
regularly consume meat are terrible at caching my son asks
my mother-in-law about a sleepover a weekend sometime
since mom and dad are fighting a lot she just changed the
subject cookie anyone? does not subscribe to the grandmother
hypothesis a parabolic rise of cases domestic and child
abuse I witness this fallout young families no support no

visitors equals no help caremongering overwhelmed lack of resource shaking yes evisceration more than once defence wounds on a four year old do you know what I do for a living? I ask him again and then cherry on top my near-immortal grandfather moves in with my uncles eliminating the only source of help we had I wake up from nightshift gobble six pieces of buttered cinnamon toast and a cold medium rare lamb chop time gets skewered so often I ask people to measure seizures in punk songs *I Wanna Be Sedated* is two minutes nineteen seconds it's been three weeks or so I guess I'm due for him to bring up divorce again I love herding dogs so smart yes but more so keen body language readers probably didn't need a puppy to the overwhelm right now though I'll give him that one a guaranteed hour almost alone every day the layers of noise not loud necessarily but ingratiating boils up something cortisol probably what I wouldn't do for some silence which is apparently a construct of the hearing but it sublimates into anger anyhow I've got a low snarl and some deep shame how often I've been yelling at my kids over nothing it's the opposite of skin hunger weighty layers of sound and presence the other mothers whisper same here when the oldest son starts compulsively washing his hands twice through the alphabet every time is distressed at interruption is washing again after touching his own face at home again after holding almost anything tries to use elbows instead washes again every ten to twenty minutes until his hands turn red and bleed clinical so hard to get my worries out as anything but stern instead of compassion a crisp and skeletal pothos hangs from the skylight dead since December it's not alone looks like it's takeout again tonight a more virulent strain begins to dominate but I can't maintain any panic this long getting laissez-faire about the yellow gowns but my spouse still can't get a vaccine the children get sore throats trouble swallowing fever and curiously red eyes however they are experienced in negotiating their swab-bribe price false alarm only costs me a

cake-pop and Pokèmon cards another virus that forever
lives in my face nests in the trigeminal nerve only shows up
under extreme physiologic stress normally only every couple
years or so keeps trying to turn my lips and eyelids whole
face on occasion into swaths of weeping blisters the
antivirals not entirely effective this time household strata of
debris laundry on underused furniture another aspect of no
visitor refrain silt up accumulation on shift I keep entering
other people's homes now the whole family gets sick by
degrees which is new actually people feel awful still have
to care for others there is no one else we checked vitals
oxygen saturation mainly we can take her alone no visitor
refrain doesn't need oxygen they send her back by cab more
contacts call back when she starts working harder to breath
triage often discharges directly from stretcher the coroner
issues death certificates a statement now these people we
often assessed suddenly dying hours later a lot to shoulder
liability our function is not should never be gatekeepers of
health care we are awaiting medical direction a directive it
is never enacted despite a field hospital erected adjacent
our hospital there is no one left to staff it in a dream I schedule
my own medically assisted death casually as a dentist
appointment somewhere between six and seventeen times a
day I receive a text for available overtime shifts it asks me to
reply "read" so I pick up a book instead unless it's a
vaccine clinic one that doesn't have plexiglass or has cut
cotton balls in half but won't turn you away for no health
card should have several translators and speakers blaring
music for the lineup around the block because an
appointment is a barrier other times a public health nurse
and myself in a spare bedroom of a rooming house these
days the most positive I've had in months great COVID
denier filter everyone wears a mask properly even my spouse
gets jabbed my mother quits her hospital job instead my son
is assigned a project on community helpers he chooses
parks and rec he asks if there are any courses I could take to

be a better mom? In May spouse and I bristle a record
length of time apathetic Mother's Day the youngest gifts me
a stone a bit rough but a good weight thick thighs save
lives I request Feist's *Metals* on the turntable oh the we're
fighting record he says makes some excellent waffles in spite
of it insert elder millennial laugh-cry emojis and side parts
here I propose framing an apartment door to the
basement he offers to not work every day I'm off making
it impossible to save first and last a well-meaning friend
asks if I wouldn't have preferred a situation where I could be
home making art I'm no good at stay-at-home I love my
family more with some space my own mother shows up two
hours late for the overpriced local brunch besides I could
never accept that amount of vulnerability speaking of my
dad comes for the weekend he and my husband soundproof
and vapour barrier the shed into a studio quiet with a
deadlock of own's own no visitors refrain he calls it my habitat
the neighbour's kid makes a COVID piñata red paper spike
proteins aerosolized candy case counts plummeting I
watch a beautiful man rollerblading though an abandoned
financial district no out-of-town visitors at midnight
gracefully he jumps and spins fully in his body and I try
care-giving again

An Unconventional Conclusion

ARUNDHATI DHARA and SARAH FRASER

Writing the conclusion of this book was tricky. After all, the book is about a pandemic that was ongoing when we wrote it. More than two years in, we are all more tired than we could have ever imagined. Reading these reflections and sitting with the art in this anthology is productively disconcerting. On one hand, there is a sense of testimony. Experiences of the first waves of COVID are laid out for everyone to read and see with us. We were not—and are not—alone. On the other hand, there is a remembering of the sense of dread, fear, and uncertainty we all shared—especially early on, when there were no vaccines and we understood so little. Many of us who worked with patients, regardless of whether they had COVID-19 or not, were sincerely afraid we might die. We promptly consulted lawyers if we didn't have wills in place, making sure our affairs were in order. We told our loved ones what to do if we got very sick, imparting to them what our children's favourite bedtime songs were, the special recipe for their birthday cake.

Just in case. Just in case?

In some ways, we have only really understood those feelings in retrospect, as we have been pushing through the daily grind of caring for patients and community.

On yet a third hand (forgive us, we are physicians, and in our work, we have often felt having three hands would be extremely helpful), experiencing these reflections is an exercise in defiance. Health-care workers went to work every day and many have not stopped since the start of the pandemic. Unexpectedly (or predictably, depending on who you ask), we have found ourselves inside a health-care system that has been revealed as incredibly fragile, a system that has left many of us looking for a way out. It is not clear whether our colleagues who want to leave health care are seeking a way out of the pandemic or care work more generally. To borrow an oft used diagnostic phrase, "it's likely multifactorial."

As we write this, we are keenly aware that "we went to work" veers dangerously close to "health-care hero" territory. We hope this book has challenged that dangerous, tired narrative. But if there is a health-care hero to be had, perhaps it is Dr. Li Wenliang (1986–2020), the whistleblower who alerted the world to what COVID-19 would mean, and who was humiliated and censured by his government before he succumbed to COVID himself (Nie and Elliott 2020). We make no such claims for ourselves. We live and work in unceded Mik'ma'ki (Nova Scotia), and like Shane's experiences as a medical trainee during 9/11 in Newfoundland, we have been spared the horrors of field hospitals and refrigeration truck morgues. But there are still So Many Patients To See. They just seemed to keep on coming, "collateral damage" in what has felt like an endless COVID wave.

"Because of COVID." This has become an answer (or excuse) for every question of "Why hasn't...?" or "Shouldn't this be...?" for seemingly every patient. We are scapegoating COVID to explain every bad outcome we see. And that's a cop out. COVID only exposed the unacceptable cracks that were already there—breaking our systems, and sometimes those within them.

This is especially true for those who were already invisible. A good portion of clinicians work with the elderly, or disenfranchised, and the care of these members of our community has long been in crisis. It's just that we had managed to avoid talking about it. COVID made it impossible to look away.

For a long time, the "infirm" (a term we'll use to capture anyone who doesn't fit neatly into a normative vision of a "productive member of society") have been presented as a monolith. They were not individuals with real personalities and desires who are deserving of care. They were nothing but the care they received. Never mind that in many cases, they have lived through catastrophes far worse than COVID and found their way through them. Many of the works in this collection are explicit about who they are and the ways COVID affected them, as a kind of resistance against such a characterization. Similarly, the hero narrative of "front-line clinicians," as perhaps society's "most productive" members during the pandemic, blunted our real humanity. We are nothing but the care we provide? Through this collection these two groups—caregivers and those being cared for—are connected. We are all revealed as infirm, productive, and whole persons.

There's a French expression "*plus ça change*," which comes from French writer Jean-Baptiste Alphonse Karr. In 1849 he wrote, "*plus ça change, plus c'est la même chose*"—the more things change, the more they stay the same. Most of the contributions in this anthology were written in 2020, in the early stages of the pandemic. At the time, we had nothing but fear, fuelled by social media feeds with images of physicians in ski masks, and dire warnings delivered by exhausted nurses with N95 imprints tattooed on their faces.

In mid-2022, at the time of writing this unconventional conclusion about a yet-to-be-concluded pandemic, we have a world with vaccines and therapeutics. We know more about interventions that help to prevent transmission. The latest variant, omicron, is widespread, but most cases are mild. Many of us have even had it. We have lifted our restrictions, and generally, we have moved on.

Yet there is an ongoing, relentless wave of secondary consequences of the pandemic we had only the vaguest inkling of as the first waves took us entirely by surprise. The opioid crisis became yet more horrifying, with death rates doubling in some regions (Palisi et al. 2021). People lost their childcare services, jobs, and incomes, and the toxic health effects of poverty became more acute. People could not (or sometimes would not) access routine care, leading to delayed diagnoses and death. Watching someone die a bad death (there's really no other way to put it), it's difficult not to think "if only..." The secret of medicine is that we can only infrequently prevent death itself. What we can do well is provide dignity and care and support a good quality of life until death comes.

Health-care workers are, in fact, just members of the population, so we aren't exempt from any of the effects we are seeing on our patients. In what is perhaps the least surprising (and endlessly discussed) repercussion of the COVID-19 pandemic, health-care workers are burned out (Canadian Medical Association 2022). Even with more information about the disease and therapeutic options, our mental health is worsening. Staff shortages are a problem across the nation, particularly in the caregiving sector. Like we said, people are looking for a way out. Not so heroic after all, but perhaps at least understandable.

The anxiety of the first waves, captured by the contributors, has not really abated. In fact, all that new information is part of the problem. The World Health Organization (2020) describes an "infodemic" as "an overabundance of information—some accurate and some not—occurring during an epidemic." They elaborate by saying an infodemic makes finding trustworthy information quite challenging. Anti-science conspiracy theories and truly bizarre notions of human physiology and virology are everywhere. We try to explain the science over and over again, even though all the data tells us that facts don't make any difference when someone's views are entrenched (Mercier and Sperber 2017). And it is exhausting.

But physicians have nothing to feel smug about. We are using Twitter feeds for treatment guidance and second-guessing public health advice with our own casual internet searches. In a way, this is no different than the public espousing clearly false theories of Ivermectin remedies that a family member came across on a podcast because it seemed to make sense.

We're a mess.

This book has captured the messy thoughts and feelings of health-care providers at a chaotic moment in history. The creativity and emotion in *The COVID Journals* will live on as a snapshot of a very specific time. The pandemic has probably changed us all to some extent. For better or for worse? For better *and* for worse.

It sometimes feels to us like the way forward is to forget. As restrictions have fallen, masks are abandoned, and people move about more freely, it's almost—*almost*—like it never happened at all. Things are "back to normal," whatever that means. But make no mistake, there's nothing new or normal about COVID-19. We know that more waves may come, new variants are possible, and we may find ourselves right back in the uncertainty of March 2020.

Plus ça change.

In Japanese culture there is an ancient art called Kintsugi. When there is damage to a piece of pottery, the broken part is repaired with gold, thus making the item stronger and more beautiful than before. In a 2022 article published in *Canadian Family Physician*, Dr. Patricia Dobkin explores the concept of the "kintsugi mind," proposing that clinicians can emerge from the pandemic stronger than before. We hope this book is part of healing the fissures that the pandemic has caused, or at least, that in its honest remembering, our fissured minds can be reassured we weren't imagining everything.

If Dr. Dobson is right, then perhaps Karr was wrong after all. We're different now. We can't go back, not exactly. Just in case, we'll take our experiences with us.

References

Canadian Medical Association. 2022. "Physician Burnout Nearly Doubles during Pandemic." News release. March 23, 2022. https://www.cma.ca/news-releases-and-statements/physician-burnout-nearly-doubles-during-pandemic.

Dobkin, Patricia Lynn. 2022. "Kintsugi Mind: How Clinicians Can Be Restored Rather than Broken by the Pandemic." *Canadian Family Physician* 68 (4): 252–54. https://doi.org/10.46747/cfp.6804252.

Mercier, Hugo, and Dan Sperber. 2017. *The Enigma of Reason*. Cambridge, MA: Harvard University Press.

Nie, Jing-Bao, and Carl Elliott. 2020. "Humiliating Whistle-Blowers: Li Wenliang, the Response to COVID-19, and the Call for a Decent Society." *Journal of Bioethical Inquiry* 17 (4): 543–47. https://doi.org/10.1007/s11673-020-09990-x.

Palisi, Heather, Marc-André Bélair, Kevin Hui, Andrew Tu, Jane Buxton, and Amanda Slaunwhite. 2021. "Overdose Deaths and the COVID-19 Pandemic in British Columbia, Canada." *Drug and Alcohol Review* 41 (4): 912–17. http//:doi.org/10.1111/dar.13424.

World Health Organization. 2020. "1st WHO Infodemiology Conference." June 30–July 16, 2020. https://www.who.int/news-room/events/detail/2020/06/30/default-calendar/1st-who-infodemiology-conference.

Acknowledgements

SHANE: Other than Damian Tarnopolsky, who was already thanked in the preface, as well as co-editors Arundhati and Sarah, I would like to thank the contributors, first and foremost; after this, the welcoming home we found at the University of Alberta Press with Michelle Lobkowicz leading the way; and trailing these thanks, I would like to offer sincere gratitude to the nascent health humanities infrastructure in Canada that has made a book like this possible. Somewhere out there, somewhen, may there be a graduate-level program in the health humanities producing the scholars that Canada desperately needs now to renovate the discipline of medicine from within. Oh, one last thanks. I renovate my list such that you are the most important. Thank you for reading.

SARAH: There are many people, places, and things that have made it possible for me to combine writing and medicine. Let's start with people. Mom, Dad, Lua, Hali, Jody, and my five siblings for being 100 per cent supportive 100 per cent of the time. My grandfather was always adamant that I write, even in the busiest moments of medicine. There were several physicians who encouraged my writing—Ron, Nick, Wendy, Bijon, and Gerri—thanks for fostering my "outside-the-box" thinking. Aruna and Shane have taught me so much and continue to do so. And University of Alberta Press—you are facilitating stories that need to be told. As for places and things, Grandpa's camp in Merigomish has given me inspiration. And finally, I'd like to thank coffee, my favourite fuel.

ARUNDHATI: To avoid that Oscar moment when the loud music starts and the winner is ushered off stage so they just stop thanking everyone they've ever met, I'll keep this brief. There is no start except to mention by name the people who make my life possible, Venkataramasastry Dhara, Malini Dhara, and Dan Rosenblum (and our three small Mango Monsters). The work of the contributors, my COVID co-editors Shane and Sarah, and my Humanities co-directors Wendy Stewart and Sarah (again) have shown me how to think bigger and better, and the kindness of Michelle Lobkowicz and University of Alberta Press in answering all my ridiculous questions is so appreciated. It's been a long road to thinking of myself as someone who writes, and all of these fine humans have pushed me along. ధన్యవాదములు

Contributors

EWAN AFFLECK is a physician who was born and raised in Montreal, and has lived and worked in northern Canada for thirty years. A nationally recognized digital health informatics expert, he lectures widely on topics such as virtual care and digital health governance and balances work in digital health policy with a part-time clinical practice. He is the executive producer and co-writer of *The Unforgotten* (2021), an award-winning film about inequities in health service for Indigenous people living in Canada. In 2013 he was appointed to the Order of Canada for his contribution to northern health care. Ewan is happily married and a father to two wonderful children.

SARAH-TAÏSSIR BENCHARIF is a physician, journalist, and writer. Her work has appeared in *Politico*, *The Globe and Mail*, *Toronto Star*, and *The Walrus*, amongst other places. She practices emergency and family medicine primarily in rural and remote Canada. She splits her time between these parts of Canada and Brussels, Belgium.

MANISHA BHARADIA is an East Indian Canadian woman born and raised in Calgary, Alberta. She is a postgraduate year-one pediatrics resident at the University of Alberta. Manisha is an avid writer and created OBLIQUITY—U of A's first humanities and medicine workshop series—with a vision to highlight the essential interconnectedness of the arts and sciences and the power of communication.

CHRISTOPHER BLAKE is a palliative care physician and writer living in Peterborough, Ontario. His academic interests include narrative medicine and public health approaches to palliative care. He writes mostly science fiction and fantasy and has a few short stories published. He also writes stories and essays in the medical humanities.

CANDACE DE TAEYE recently completed her MFA in creative writing at the University of Guelph. Her poetry has been published in *Arc*, *BAD NUDES*, *Carousel*, *CNQ*, *CV2*, *Grain*, *Vallum,* and others. Her most recent collection of poetry *Pronounced / Workable* was published in 2022 by Mansfield Press. During the day, and more often at night, she works as a paramedic in Toronto's downtown core. She lives in Guelph with her partner, kids, some geriatric tree frogs, and a twenty-five-pound tortoise.

ARUNDHATI DHARA is a family physician in Mi'kma'ki (Nova Scotia) and co-director of the Medical Humanities Program at Dalhousie University. She studied liberal arts and public health, but her heart really lies at the intersections of identity, family, and medicine for physicians and the public. She would find more time to write if not for her three small monsters, who seem to suck up all the moments of the day.

PAUL DHILLON is a writer and physician from British Columbia. His most recent publication is *The Surprising Lives of Small-Town Doctors*, a compilation of rural physician stories from across Canada that captures the challenges and magic of working as a rural physician. Previous writing received the 2011 Aindreas McEntee Prize presented by the Irish Association of Medical Writers and he was recognized as a New England Journal of Medicine Scholar in the 200th Anniversary Dialogues in Medicine Essay Competition. "The Viral Hospital," detailing experiences in the Kerry Town Ebola Treatment Centre, was recently published in *Emergency Medicine Narratives: An Emergency Medicine Humanities Collection.*

LIAM DURCAN is a neurologist who works at the McGill University Health Centre. He is the author of two novels, *Garcia's Heart* and *The Measure of Darkness*, and a collection of short stories titled *A Short Journey by Car*.

MONIKA DUTT is the daughter of immigrants of South Asian ancestry and a settler on Unama'ki (Cape Breton, Nova Scotia). She is a specialist in public health and preventive medicine and the Medical Officer of Health for Central and Western Newfoundland and Labrador. She is also a family physician at the Ally Centre of Cape Breton and a member of the Decent Work and Health Network. She sees elements of stories in the people and places she encounters, and finds writing a way to explore those stories.

SARAH FRASER is a general practitioner working in Mi'kma'ki (Nova Scotia). She is also associate editor/humanities at *Canadian Family Physician* and co-director of the Medical Humanities Program at Dalhousie University Medical School. She believes it is meaningful to incorporate story into the practice of medicine, and life.

DAVID GRATZER is a Toronto-based psychiatrist and physician. He works at the Centre for Addiction and Mental Health, where he is an attending psychiatrist, and serves as the co-chief of the General Adult Psychiatry and Health Systems Division. He is active in teaching, and recently won the Peter Selby Award for Excellence in Technology-Enhanced Education. He has been nominated ten times for University of Toronto teaching awards. He peer reviews for several journals, including *CMAJ*, and he sits on the editorial board of *JMIR Mental Health*; he is an associate editor of the *Canadian Journal of Psychiatry*.

JILLIAN HORTON is an associate professor of internal medicine at the University in Manitoba. She is a regular contributor to the *LA Times* and *The Globe and Mail*; her work appears by syndication in a number of US newspapers. Her first book, *We Are All Perfectly Fine: A Memoir of Love, Medicine and Healing*, was published by HarperCollins Canada in February 2021 and is a national bestseller.

ANDREW HOWE, ANGELA E. SIMMONDS, BOBBY TAYLOR, DOLLY WILLIAMS, and CHADWICK WILLIAMS are from the African Nova Scotian communities of North Preston, East Preston, and Cherry Brook. They are leaders, advocates and activists in their communities.

MONICA KIDD has written several books of poetry, fiction, nonfiction and poetry, most recently *Chance Encounters with Wild Animals* (Gaspereau Press, 2019). Formerly a staff reporter with CBC Radio, she works as a freelance journalist and practices family medicine with low-risk obstetrics in Alberta and Newfoundland and Labrador. She is an associate editor of humanities at the *CMAJ*.

JAIME LENET is a hospital social worker, a PHD candidate, and the mother of two young children. She has taught social work and social policy to students at two universities and has close to twenty years of experience working in community and institutional settings. Jaime is consistently frustrated by the contradictory nature of seeking social justice from within economic and political systems built upon oppression. She often finds herself heartbroken, guilt-ridden, and enraged by her work in health and education, and by her research into Canada's removal of former refugee claimants.

PAM LENKOV is an educator and clinician in Toronto at Sunnybrook Health Sciences Centre, and at Women's College Hospital where she is the director of Undergraduate Medical Education. She is an assistant professor in the Department of Family and Community Medicine at the University of Toronto. She strongly believes that medicine is not only a science but also an art that, if nurtured, lends itself to narrative expression.

SUZANNE LILKER is an anaesthesiologist at St. Joseph's Health Centre and assistant professor at University of Toronto. She is also a student of narrative medicine, with an interest in emotional intelligence and wellness. She is single mother to a daughter and a Portuguese water dog. Experiences and observations during COVID times have made her more aware of the human condition, our frailty, and her own vulnerability, and motivated her to write the poem included in this collection.

JENNIFER MOORE is a palliative medicine physician at Sunnybrook Health Sciences Centre in Toronto, Ontario. She is an associate professor in the Division of Palliative Medicine/Department of Medicine at the University of Toronto. Jennifer is originally from Chicago, but lives in Toronto with her husband and three children, where she also serves as a butler for their Newfoundland dog, Jones.

SHANE NEILSON is a poet and physician from New Brunswick. He has published several books of poetry, non-fiction, and fiction, including the affect trilogy from Porcupine's Quill (*Complete Physical*, *On Shaving*, and *Dysphoria*). He is an adjunct professor of family medicine at the Waterloo Regional Campus of McMaster University and has a special interest in the mental health of adolescents and young adults. His most recent book is *You May Not Take the Sad and Angry Consolations* from Goose Lane Editions (2022), a text that engages with lived experience of neurodiversity.

KACPER NIBURSKI is a resident in anesthesia at the University of British Columbia, a twin-wannabe-triplet, and a wobbly writer. He has been published in *JAMA*, *CMAJ*, and others. You can find his work either in the garbage, or occasionally, on his Instagram: @_kenkan.

ELIZABETH NIEDRA is a writer and home-based care of the elderly physician in Toronto, Ontario, and a lecturer in the Department of Family and Community Medicine at the University of Toronto. Her work has appeared in *Canadian Family Physician*, *CBC Opinions,* and the *Button Eye Review.* She lives in Toronto with her partner and two dogs.

MARGARET NOWACZYK is a pediatric clinical geneticist. Her short stories and essays have appeared in Canadian, American, and Polish literary magazines and her memoir, *Chasing Zebras*, was published in 2021. She lives in Hamilton, Ontario, with her husband and two sons.

TOLU OLORUNTOBA is the author of two full-length collections of poetry: *The Junta of Happenstance* and *Each One a Furnace.* After a somewhat itinerant life in Nigeria and the United States, he emigrated to the Greater Vancouver Area, where he lives with his family and manages projects for health organizations.

RORY O'SULLIVAN is a family physician in Toronto. He has had the opportunity to practice in rural communities and urban centres across four provinces, and to collect extraordinary stories along the way. He is passionate about Indigenous health and the care of vulnerable populations. His narrative work has previously been published in *Intima: A Journal of Narrative Medicine.* He was the recipient of the 2022 College of Family Physicians of Canada Mimi Divinsky Award for History and Narrative in Family Medicine.

JORDAN PELC is a hospitalist physician working at Sinai Health in Toronto, and an assistant professor in the Department of Family and Community Medicine in the Temerty Faculty of Medicine at the University of Toronto.

NICK PIMLOTT is a family physician and writer in Toronto. He is the scientific editor of *Canadian Family Physician* and a professor in the Department of Family and Community Medicine, Temerty Faculty of Medicine, University of Toronto.

TANAS SYLLIBOY is from Eskasoni First Nation in Nova Scotia. They are a Mi'kmaw nurse practitioner working in the Mi'kmaw community of Millbrook. They also work in the field of pediatric emergency care and pain research, looking at ways to transform pediatric care for Indigenous populations. In 2021 Tanas was awarded the Dr. Robert Strang Community Hero Award, which recognized their devotion and commitment to keeping people safe in Mi'kma'ki during the pandemic. One worldview they think we can all benefit from is the concept/word *Apoqnmatulti'k*, meaning "we help each other."

HELEN TANG is a medical student at the University of Saskatchewan. She obtained her undergraduate degree in physiology and pharmacology and is now hoping to pursue a career in rural family medicine. In her spare time, she loves to paint, ski, practice yoga, mountain bike, and rock climb. She would like to include her love for art and physical activity into her family medicine practice through obtaining a fellowship in integrative medicine. Helen would like to thank Dr. Tom Rosenal and Heather Huston from the University of Calgary for their guidance and counselling.

THARSHIKA THANGARASA is a daughter, sister, friend, aspiring artist, and psychiatry resident at the University of Toronto. The COVID-19 pandemic has created a collective chaos that has swept across the globe. Like many others, she floundered to try and create meaning amidst a situation with so many unknowns and moving parts. Ultimately, she rediscovered art as a tool to process emotions and create pieces that others can (hopefully) resonate with. This pandemic has challenged our norms, relationships, and even our perceived safety. However, in bringing us together through shared experience, she hopes art can make it a little easier.

DIANA TOUBASSI is an assistant professor and clinician-teacher at the University of Toronto Department of Family and Community Medicine. Her clinical practice is based at the University Health Network–Toronto Western Hospital, where she served as postgraduate director for eight years. Her academic interests include physician well-being, professional identity formation and evolution, and psychology and narrative. Her most recent efforts focus on exploring the contribution of professional identity to trainee wellness. Dr. Toubassi's work has been supported by several education scholarship awards, and she has disseminated her work in a number of publications and conference presentations.

SHAN WANG is a Chinese Canadian in Montreal, sharing her experience as a certified nursing assistant in an understaffed nursing home during the first wave of COVID-19. She has since been working as a registered nurse and pursuing her bachelor of nursing (integrated) (BNI) degree at McGill University. Shan is currently the internal communication coordinator for the McGill Association of Students in Healthcare. She has also co-founded the McGill Mentorships in Healthcare for under-represented Collège d'enseignement général et professionnel (CEGEP, general and vocational college) students. When she can, Shan enjoys hiking in nature, writing, and painting.

MARISA WEBSTER is a public health and preventative medicine resident at the University of Alberta. She has a master of arts in philosophy and is currently working on a master of public health. Her work is published in *Frontier Poetry*, *Open Minds Quarterly*, *Peculiars Magazine*, *Canadian Family Physician*, and the *Dalhousie Medical Journal*. She was long-listed in the Palette Poetry Emerging Poet Prize Competition in 2021 and is a contributor to the anthology *Wonder Shift*. She has slung coffee for a living, busted her ankle rock climbing, and swigged Pepsi Blue on a houseboat in Kashmir. In addition to writing, she is a dedicated yoga practitioner, voracious reader, avid photographer, and lover of laughter. She believes that healing comes in many forms.

JIAMENG XU graduated from the MD-PHD program at McGill University in 2021. She completed her PHD dissertation, "Practices of Being Near: An Ethnographic Study of Family Members and Persons with Lived Experience of Mental Illness," in the department of Rehabilitation Science and the Connected Narratives Lab led by Professor Melissa Park. She completed undergraduate studies in life sciences, concentrating in neuroscience, at Queen's University in Kingston, Ontario. She has been involved in initiatives to create a space for the arts and humanities within health professional training and settings of health-care delivery. Currently a psychiatry resident at the University of British Columbia, she aims to dedicate her career to working with patients and their families.

Other Titles from University of Alberta Press

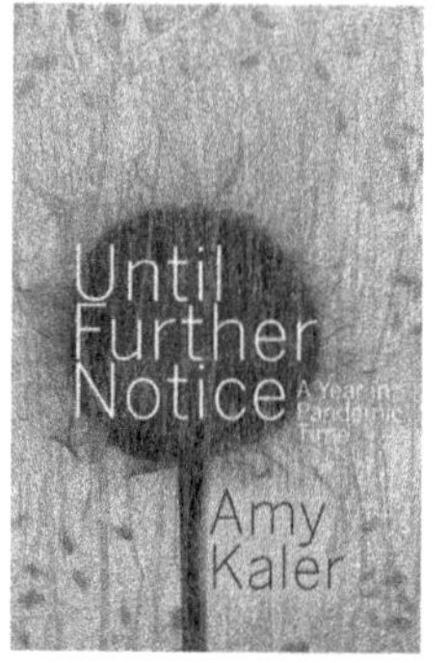

UNTIL FURTHER NOTICE

A Year in Pandemic Time

AMY KALER

Amy Kaler explores the changing consciousness and confusion of life during the COVID-19 pandemic's first year. Reflexive and relatable, she captures fine-grained, everyday experiences from an extraordinary year.

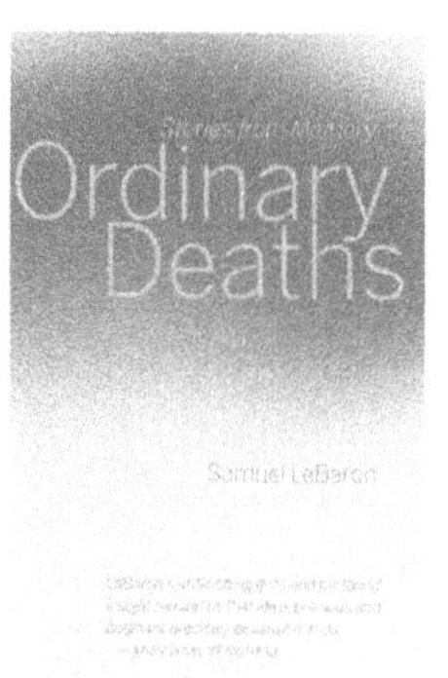

ORDINARY DEATHS

Stories from Memory

SAMUEL LEBARON

Dr. Samuel LeBaron reminds us of our need for human connection when experiencing death and loss. Based on over thirty years of working with children and adults dying from cancer, LeBaron's memoir contains stories of longing, confusion, love, and humility, helping readers find solace and confidence.

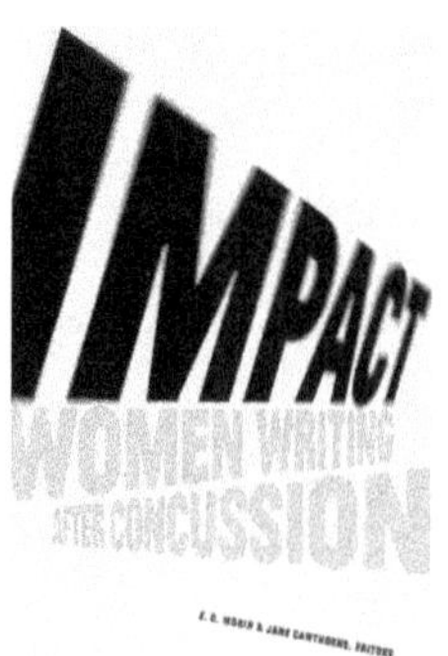

IMPACT

Women Writing After Concussion

Edited by E.D. MORIN & JANE CAWTHORNE

Twenty-one women writers consider the effects of concussion on their personal and professional lives and offer vital counter-narratives to "one-size-fits-all" descriptions of traumatic brain injuries and recovery.

More information at uap.ualberta.ca

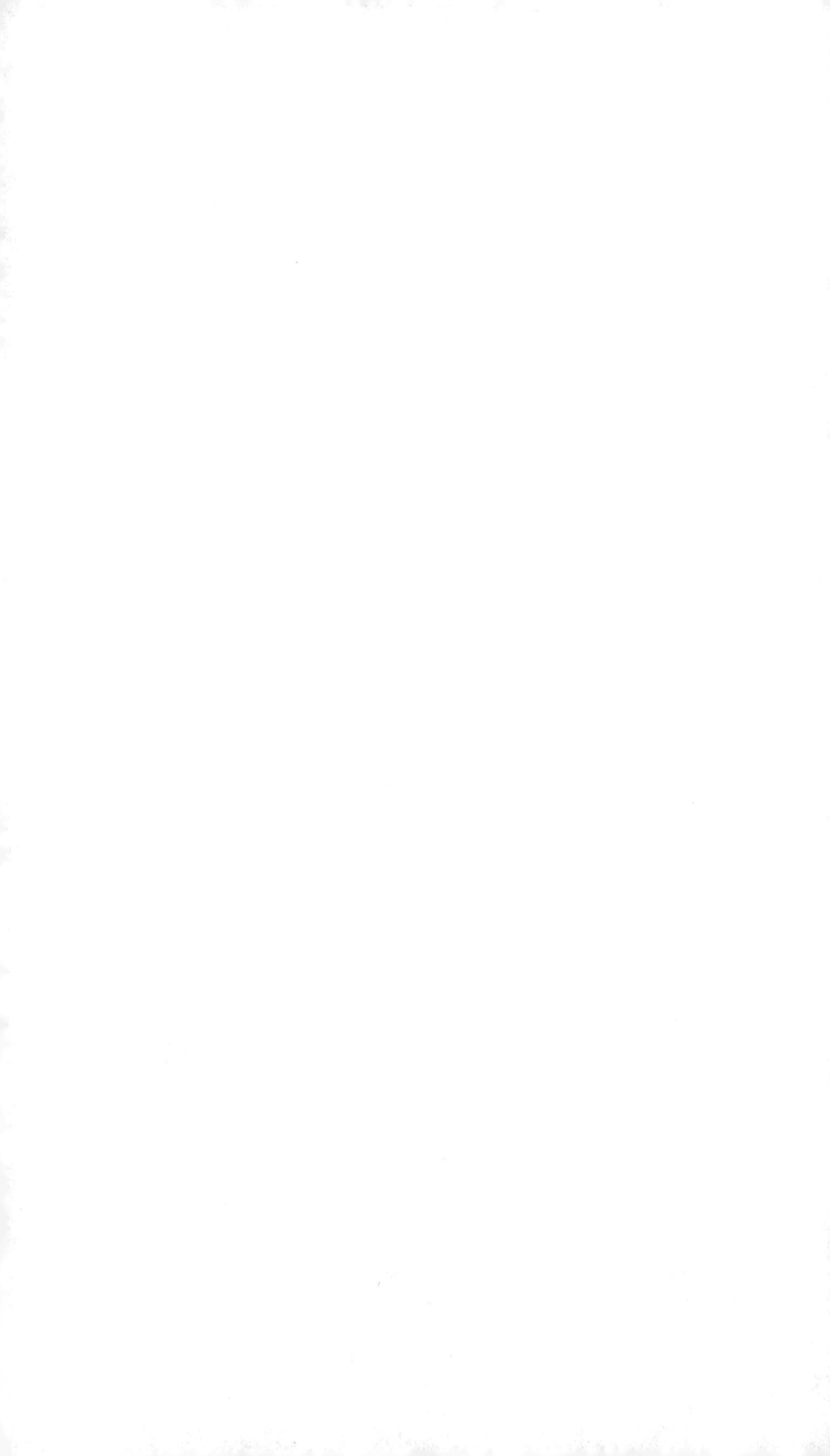

www.ingramcontent.com/pod-product-compliance
Lightning Source LLC
Chambersburg PA
CBHW020319211224
19360CB00002B/3

9 781772 12681